About the Authors

Gillian Hotz, Ph.D., CCC-SLP, is the Co-director of the Pediatric Brain & Spinal Cord Injury Program; Director of Neurotrauma Outcome Research, Concussion, and WalkSafe Programs; and Associate Research Professor in the Department of Neurosurgery at the University of Miami Miller School of Medicine, Miami, Florida. Dr. Hotz is Principal Investigator on a variety of funded research projects for acute care and rehabilitation of children with traumatic brain injury and injury prevention. She has presented at local, national, and international conferences; has published numerous papers on the topic of traumatic brain injury; and is coauthor of the *Brief Test of Head Injury* (with Nancy Helm-Estabrooks, PRO-ED, 1991). Dr. Hotz is a member of a number of advisory groups, including the Florida Injury Prevention Advisory Council and the Sarah Jane Brain Project/The National Pediatric Acquired Brain Injury Plan.

Nancy Helm-Estabrooks, Sc.D., CCC-SLP, is the Caroline Brewer Smith Distinguished Professor in the Department of Communication Disorders and Sciences at Western Carolina University in Cullowhee, North Carolina. She was affiliated with the Harold Goodglass Aphasia Research Center and Boston University School of Medicine for 32 years, was a Research Scientist at the National Center for Neurogenic Communication Disorders at The University of Arizona, and was a Research Professor at the University of North Carolina, where she retains an adjunct position. Dr. Helm-Estabrooks is board certified by the Academy of Neurologic Communication Disorder (ANCDS). Her awards include American Speech-Language-Hearing Association (ASHA) and ANCDS Honors. She is an ASHA fellow and has published more than 90 peer-reviewed articles, 7 books, 21 chapters, and 6 standardized tests.

Nickola Wolf Nelson, Ph.D., CCC-SLP, is Professor in the Department of Speech Pathology and Audiology and Director of the Ph.D. program in Interdisciplinary Health Sciences at Western Michigan University in Kalamazoo. She also serves as Editor of *Topics in Language Disorders*. She has been working for the past 35 years providing services and conducting research related to language and literacy development and disorders in childhood. Dr. Nelson has published numerous journal articles, chapters, and books, including *Language and Literacy Disorders: Infancy through Adolescence* (Allyn & Bacon, 2010). Dr. Nelson is a fellow of the American Speech-Language-Hearing Association and the International Academy of Learning Disabilities. In 2007, she received the Frank R. Kleffner Clinical Career Award.

Pediatric Test of Brain Injury™ PTBI™
Examiner's Manual

Other components of the Pediatric Test of Brain Injury™
Test Form
Stimulus Book

Pediatric Test of Brain Injury™ PTBI™
Examiner's Manual

by

Gillian Hotz, Ph.D., CCC-SLP
University of Miami Miller School of Medicine
Miami, Florida

Nancy Helm-Estabrooks, Sc.D., CCC-SLP
Western Carolina University
Cullowhee, North Carolina

Nickola Wolf Nelson, Ph.D., CCC-SLP
Western Michigan University
Kalamazoo

and

Elena Plante, Ph.D., CCC-SLP
The University of Arizona
Tucson

PAUL H. BROOKES PUBLISHING CO.®

Baltimore • London • Sydney

Paul H. Brookes Publishing Co.
Post Office Box 10624
Baltimore, Maryland 21285-0624
USA

www.brookespublishing.com

Typeset by Spearhead Global, Inc., Bear, Delaware.
Manufactured in China by JADE PRODUCTIONS.

Library of Congress Cataloging-in-Publication Data

Pediatric test of brain injury (PTBI) examiner's manual / by Gillian Hotz ... [et al.].
p. ; cm.
Includes bibliographical references and index.
ISBN-13: 978-1-59857-111-0 (pbk.)
ISBN-10: 1-59857-111-7 (pbk.)
1. Brain-damaged children. 2. Neuropsychological tests for children. I. Hotz, Gillian. II. Title.
[DNLM: 1. Brain Injuries—diagnosis. 2. Child. 3. Neuropsychological Tests. WS 340 P37185 2010]
RJ496.B7P434 2010
618.92'8—dc22 2010001815

British Library Cataloguing in Publication data are available from the British Library.

2014 2013 2012 2011 2010

10 9 8 7 6 5 4 3 2 1

Contents

Elena Plante, Ph.D., CCC-SLP, is Professor and Head of the Department of Speech, Language, and Hearing Sciences at The University of Arizona in Tucson. She is a fellow both of The University of Arizona's College of Science and of the American Speech-Language-Hearing Association. Her areas of research interest include language learning and assessment practices. Dr. Plante has been using neuroimaging to explore the brain bases of language and cognition for the last 2 decades. She has active national and international collaborations in the areas of neuroimaging, language, and learning.

Acknowledgments

We extend special thanks to the clinicians and the facilities across the United States and Canada that participated in the field testing of the PTBI and are listed here. We also are grateful for the clinicians' feedback as to the utility and usefulness of this test. The protocols they returned made it possible to bring this test to completion.

1. *Coordinating Center*—University of Miami Miller School of Medicine/Jackson Memorial Medical Center, Miami, Florida: Gillian Hotz, Ph.D.; Beth Zeldis, Psy.D.; and Sherika Colston, B.A.
2. Alberta Children's Hospital, Alberta, Canada: Shirley Leew, Ph.D.
3. Akron Children's Hospital, Akron, Ohio: Kathleen A. Considine, M.A., CCC-SLP; and Sheila Hostetler, M.A., CCC-SLP
4. Nationwide Children's Hospital, Columbus, Ohio: Jennifer Lundine, M.A., CCC-SLP; and Stephanie Oswald, M.A., CCC-SLP
5. Children's Healthcare of Atlanta, Atlanta, Georgia: Julie Haarbauer-Krupa, Ph.D., CCC-SLP
6. The Montreal Children's Hospital, Montreal, Québec, Canada: Katrine Doucet, M.Sc.(A), S-LP(C); and Isabelle Gagnon, Ph.D.
7. National Rehabilitation Hospital, Washington, D.C.: Brownrigg Snow, M.S., CCC-SLP; and Lauren Clark, M.A., CCC-SLP
8. The Patricia Neal Rehabilitation Center at Fort Sanders Regional Medical Center, Knoxville, Tennessee: Al Kaye, M.S., CTRS; Deborah Rhyne, M.A., CCC-SLP; Michelle Rugen, M.S., CCC-SLP; and Mary Margaret Preston, M.A., CCC-SLP
9. Phoenix Children's Hospital, Phoenix, Arizona: Michael S. Lavoie, Ph.D.; and Lindsay M. Stevens, M.A., CCC-SLP
10. The Rehabilitation Institute of Kansas City, Kansas City, Missouri: Nicole Conforti, M.S., CCC-SLP
11. Rehabilitation Institute of Chicago, Chicago, Illinois: Victoria Nahmad, M.S., CCC-SLP; and Kathryn Demarco, M.S., CCC-SLP
12. St. Louis Children's Hospital, St. Louis, Missouri: Mary Warburton, M.A., CCC-SLP; and Casey Stallings, M.S., CCC-SLP

13. St. Joseph's Hospital and Medical Center/Barrow Neurological Institute, Phoenix, Arizona: Sharon Duckwiler, M.A., CCC-SLP; and Jana Thompson, M.N.S., CCC-SLP

14. University of North Carolina Hospitals, Chapel Hill, North Carolina: Leah MacMillan, M.S., CCC-SLP

In addition, we thank the Feder Family and their friends for assisting with subject recruitment and Anabel Anon for all of her work with the test database.

The development and publication of the PTBI would not have been possible without the early contributions of Tom Hutchinson and recent contributions of Paul H. Brookes Publishing Co., Inc. As authors, we extend our heartfelt thanks to all of those who have made the publication of this test possible.

To all those children and adolescents who have sustained a traumatic or other form of acquired brain injury. We hope that the PTBI will be helpful in assessing their neurocognitive and language skills and needs and will lead to effective recommendations for treatment and reintegration into their schools and communities.

1

Introduction

A NEW KIND OF TEST

The Pediatric Test of Brain Injury™ (PTBI™) is not like other tests—and it shouldn't be. The PTBI was built specifically to address the assessment needs of children and adolescents with brain injuries. The unique needs of these individuals demanded that we develop a new kind of test.

The two major purposes of testing children with brain injury are to establish current ability levels and to track changes over time. To accomplish these goals, it is important to obtain the most accurate estimate of ability possible from performance on the test. Most tests estimate ability by having the examiner count the number of items passed; the more items passed, the more ability is assumed on the child's part. Unfortunately, this approach ignores the fact that the difficulty of test items may not be evenly incremental.

Consider an example for the purpose of discussion. Imagine a three-item test; the first item on the test is very easy, the next is slightly less easy, and the third is very difficult. A child who receives a score of 2 by passing the first and second items will be considerably less able than a second child who receives a score of 2 by passing any other combination of two items. Unless the difficulty level of the items is known, it is impossible to tell the actual ability levels of these children apart. Furthermore, a "1 point/no point" estimate of ability can mask the true amount of change experienced by children as they recover. Therefore, simply assigning a point for each item passed is an ineffective and inaccurate system for assessing the needs of children with brain injuries. For the PTBI, we overcame this limitation by rethinking how to score test items.

For the PTBI, we statistically evaluated the relative difficulty of each item within each subtest using item response theory (IRT) procedures. IRT is an advanced method of evaluating test items. It permits each individual item on a test to be assigned a number that reflects how difficult that item is relative to the other items on the test. The items are scaled so that the easiest item on the test is rated at 0.5 and all other items are rated based on how much more difficult they are than the easiest item. The advantage of this method is that examiners are able to calculate an ability score for a test that reflects a child's current level of functioning more accurately than a simple count of items passed, leading to a superior ability to track change.

Additional innovative features also are incorporated within this manual. We strived to make information concise and user friendly while still addressing the relevant standards set forth in the *Standards for Educational and Psychological Testing* by the American Educational Research Association, American Psychological Association, and National Council on Measurement in Education (1999). We laid out validity and reliability information in an evidenced-based practice format so that clinicians could easily see whether data support the interpretations they want to make based on the test scores. Because this test is different in various respects from typical pediatric tests, we strongly recommend that examiners read all chapters of this manual thoroughly prior to using the test to assure that they correctly administer, score, and interpret the PTBI. We think that professionals who use the PTBI will find the test both easy to use and useful for assessing the cognitive-linguistic abilities of children with brain injury.

PURPOSE

The purpose of the PTBI is to estimate a child's ability in applying neurocognitive-linguistic skills that are vulnerable to pediatric brain injury and relevant to functioning well in school. The test is intended to permit tracking of recovery starting in the acute phase and continuing until PTBI performance indicates functioning in the mild to normal range.

OVERVIEW

The PTBI is designed to assess neurocognitive and language abilities of individuals recovering from brain injury relevant to the academic demands of school. This test is criterion-referenced and provides cut-off scores for each subtest that can be used to describe age-related ability ratings and severity classifications.

TARGET POPULATION

The PTBI is appropriate for use with children and adolescents ages 6–16 years who have sustained a traumatic brain injury (TBI) or acquired brain injury (ABI) and who represent all levels of severity. A TBI is a brain injury resulting from a traumatic event caused by an external physical force (e.g., motor vehicle crash, a fall, a sports-related injury, a gunshot wound, assault, a blast injury). The term *TBI* applies to open and closed head injuries. Open head injuries include penetrating injuries (e.g., gunshot or missile); closed head injuries occur as a result of a blow to the head in which the skull is not penetrated. Both open and closed head injuries can result in brain damage that is focal, diffuse, or widespread and can range from mild to severe. ABI is caused by nontraumatic neurological events such as a stroke, a brain tumor, a seizure disorder, encephalitis, anoxia, meningitis, inflammation, drugs, toxins, metabolic disorders, or other forms of nontraumatic brain disease.

The PTBI is designed for use with children and adolescents in acute care settings (including at the bedside) and in rehabilitation facilities and clinics. It also can be used to assess levels of performance and track change for children with brain injuries (TBI or ABI) who are at home or who have returned to school. Although the PTBI is intended for use starting in the acute phases of recovery following TBI, the PTBI should be used with caution and sensitivity when a child is in an acute confusional state or when a child is unable to attend to a structured activity for 5 minutes.

EXAMINER QUALIFICATIONS

Speech-language pathologists, psychologists, or other specialists trained to assess children and adolescents with cognitive-communication impairments, including brain injury, are qualified to administer the PTBI.

TEST ADMINISTRATION

The PTBI can be administered to children and adolescents at the bedside as well as in other hospital, clinical, home, or school settings. It can be administered in one session lasting approximately 30 minutes or in two sessions. When administration takes place over two sessions, these sessions should occur on the same day. The first session should include Subtests 1–5. The second session should include Subtests 6–10. This is essential to incorporate immediate and delayed memory subtests of the same stimuli in the same session.

TEST COMPONENTS

The test components for the PTBI include an Examiner's Manual, Stimulus Book, and Test Form. The examiner will need the Examiner's Manual to score the PTBI and obtain a performance category for each subtest.

Examiner's Manual

This Examiner's Manual provides directions for administering, scoring, and interpreting the test. It also includes information about test development, field testing, and evidence of reliability and validity along with a case example.

Stimulus Book

The spiral-bound Stimulus Book provides the visual stimuli for the subtests of Word Fluency, What Goes Together, Naming, and Yes/No/Maybe.

Test Form

Page 1 of the Test Form includes space for recording critical information about the child and the testing circumstances and for summarizing the child's performance on the test. At the top of each subtest is an instructions banner that makes key information easy to find. This key information includes materials needed for administration, what to say when instructing the child, prompts that are allowed or not, discontinue and repetition rules, and guidelines for scoring. Spaces are provided for recording children's responses to test stimuli as well as weighted *ability scores,* which are based on empirically derived item difficulty. Each subtest also includes a behavioral observations checklist and space for noting issues such as the need to refocus attention, difficulty maintaining set, and perseveration. In addition, notes for examiners are provided at the end of each subtest to highlight particularly relevant behaviors to observe for that subtest.

Other Materials

In addition to the components included in the test kit, the examiner must provide the following:

- Pen (preferably felt-tipped with black ink and a point fine enough for drawing)
- Watch with a second hand or a stopwatch that displays time in seconds
- Calculator for adding ability scores

SCORING

Scoring principles for the PTBI can be found in Chapter 5. As noted in this chapter, the PTBI is a new kind of criterion-referenced standardized test. The scoring is based on ability scores that are evidence-based. The ability scores and interpretation criteria have been derived from field testing of the standardization version (Version 2) of the PTBI. This version was constructed based on multiple research versions and pilot tests. Using age-appropriate criterion-referenced guidelines, examiners will be able to indicate whether a child, at a particular point in time, is demonstrating high performance, moderate performance, low performance, or very low performance in areas of cognitive-linguistic functioning that are known to be vulnerable to pediatric brain injury and relevant to functioning well in school. The performance categories are anchored to the scores obtained from children without brain injuries (see Chapter 6, Table 6.1). The majority of scores from children without brain injuries fall within the high performance category on all subtests, with decreasing numbers of children scoring in the categories that reflect lower performance.

CONCLUSION

The PTBI is a new kind of test to address the assessment needs of children and adolescents with brain injuries. The theoretical background and rationale for the PTBI are described in Chapter 2.

2

Theoretical Background and Rationale

The need for a standardized test to assess neurocognitive and language functioning in children and adolescents with brain injuries was highlighted in a 2003 technical report of the American Speech-Language-Hearing Association, "Rehabilitation of Children and Adults with Cognitive-Communication Disorders after Brain Injury," and in the article "Guidelines for the Acute Medical Management of Severe Traumatic Brain Injury in Infants, Children and Adolescents" (Adelson et al., 2003). According to these documents, a clinical need exists to assess current skill levels and produce objective data for tracking recovery from TBI and to justify continued inpatient and outpatient treatment services. The PTBI was developed to meet these needs (Hotz, Helm-Estabrooks, & Nelson, 2001; Hotz, Helm-Estabrooks, Nelson, & Plante, 2009).

The issue of using formal tests for early assessment of children and adolescents recovering from brain injury has been met with contrasting opinions. Ylvisaker and colleagues (2005), for example, warned against stressing patients during early recovery by administering formal tests. It should be noted, however, that as soon as children move beyond the level of confusion and/or agitation, critical information can be obtained from a brief but controlled observation of their performance. As a standardized, evidence-based instrument, the PTBI can provide critical information regarding areas of impaired and retained ability and can serve as a baseline against which to measure recovery. An additional practical need for standardized testing stems from requirements by insurance companies and others for objective data to justify the need for services.

Even though ecological, contextualized observations are invaluable to the assessment process, these often are difficult to conduct when a child is hospitalized or in a rehabilitation center. Formal tests can be designed to be administered at the bedside and in short segments. They can efficiently target skills most likely to be spared and impaired at varying levels of severity in a particular clinical population such as individuals with TBI, including those with relatively mild injuries. Some children who might demonstrate abilities that appear "normal" during naturalistic interactions may exhibit moderate performance deficits on tasks that require higher-level, integrated cognitive-linguistic processes such as those needed for academic performance.

Of critical concern in developing a test for use with pediatric populations is that it must achieve two goals in order to demonstrate construct and content validity. First, it must measure a range of developmentally appropriate abilities. Second, it must sample abilities that are of particular concern for the population of interest—in this case, children affected by TBI and ABI. Addressing both goals in a single instrument for this population presents some unusual challenges, which are discussed in the sections that follow.

CONSTRAINED AND UNCONSTRAINED DEVELOPMENTAL ABILITIES

Researchers, test designers, and statisticians face special challenges when developing tests for children and adolescents, especially those with brain injuries. Some important skills, such as communicating basic information about age, time, and place; following simple commands; and naming common objects develop fairly early in childhood and remain stable unless impaired by disease or injury. In the developmental literature, such abilities are termed *constrained* (e.g., Paris, 2005), in that they reach the top of the developmental curve fairly early, after which little variance is observed (i.e., a *ceiling effect*). Because ceiling effects begin to be noted at fairly young ages, tasks measuring constrained abilities do not work well for some types of testing (e.g., norm-referenced tests) across wider age ranges. Too little variance occurs in test scores to allow them to represent meaningful differences. That does not mean, however, that constrained abilities cannot be compromised by brain injury, making them appropriate for inclusion in criterion-referenced tests for this population. The PTBI incorporates three subtests that measure constrained abilities—Orientation, Following Commands, and Naming.

Conversely, *unconstrained* developmental abilities (Paris, 2005) develop across a wider age range and require organization and integration of abilities that cross cognitive and linguistic domains. They continue to show enough variance to capture evidence of developmental advances across a wider age span. Language comprehension and discourse formulation tasks fall into this category, as do cognitive process tasks that require people to search their memories to recall and organize bits of information into meaningful wholes. Chapman, Levin, Wanek, Weyrach, and Kufera (1998) described narrative discourse as requiring the "ability to use the language system to select, organize, and integrate information" (p. 426). Thus, narration is an example of going beyond isolated language skills to tap into the multifaceted relationships that language and cognition share. Research on the PTBI (discussed in Chapter 6) showed that most subtests performed psychometrically as unconstrained measures of developmental advances across the age range of the test.

NEUROCOGNITIVE AND LINGUISTIC SEQUELAE OF BRAIN INJURY

Pediatric brain injury consequences are complex and multifaceted. Typical areas of impairment include a wide range of deficits involving arousal, attention, perception, concentration, speed of processing, memory (immediate and delayed), language, learning, thinking, reasoning, problem solving, and executive functioning (Krichevsky, Chang, & Squire, 2004; Rao & Lyketsos, 2000; Vital, 2002). When attention, memory, and learning capacities are impaired, academic progress typically is compromised as well (Ylvisaker, 1998; Ylvisaker et al., 2005). Studies have reported difficulties involving attention, speed of processing, learning efficiency, and executive functions even for children with mild TBI (Cicerone, 1996; Raskin, Mateer, & Tweeten, 1998). Furthermore, such difficulties may persist for years, causing children with moderate and severe brain injuries to fall further and further behind their peers in academic performance (Babikian & Asarnow, 2009; Fay et al., 2009).

Moreover, because children who sustain brain injuries are in the process of developing neurocognitive and linguistic skills, age at the time of injury becomes a key factor in the assessment. The course of development after pediatric brain injury for individual children is influenced by many factors associated with intertwining factors of maturation, neuroplasticity, and the development of academic language and literacy skills through formal education. Although no test, especially a brief one, can be expected to provide both the depth and breadth of information needed to develop comprehensive rehabilitation programs, we have designed the PTBI to permit observation of the key areas of deficit that are likely to be affected following brain injury.

Attention

Attention is commonly affected in children and adolescents recovering from TBI. Attention is critical for information processing, learning, and successful execution of activities of daily living. According to Lezak, Howieson, Loring, Hannay, and Fisher (2004), "intact attention is a necessary precondition of both concentration and mental tracking activities" (p. 348). Attentional functions are frequently impaired with frontal lobe lesions, and frontal damage is a common outcome of TBI. Children with brain injury may be slow in reacting to stimuli, unable to maintain focus, and highly susceptible to distractions. From a cognitive development perspective, attention skills emerge gradually through childhood. Sustained attention matures relatively early, and other abilities, including the capacity to focus and shift attention, are acquired later as the child matures (McKay, Halperin, Schwartz, & Sharma, 1994).

Memory

Memory impairments also are commonly reported in children recovering from brain injury. Depending on the location of the brain injury, memory impairments may affect all or some of the processes involved in learning new information. Learning requires attending, receiving, processing, and integrating information (Goldstein, Len, & Boake, 1989); storing learned information (Crosson, Novack, Trenerry, & Cragi, 1988); and retrieving stored information (Wilde, Boake, & Sherer, 1995). Success in educational settings requires a student to attend to, process, integrate, store, and retrieve large amounts of information, while complexity increases across grade levels (Milton, Scaglione, Flanagan, Cox, & Rudnick, 1991). Several types of memory processes have been described in the neuropsychological literature. It has been well documented that most individuals with TBI, even those with mild TBI, have working memory impairments (Levin et al., 2004; McDowell, Whyte, & D'Esposito, 1997). Children in the acute stages of recovery also may have difficulty remembering events of the day or what they do in therapy sessions, which is described as *episodic memory* (Levin et al., 1996).

Language

Although language ability is not consistently impaired following brain injury, several aspects of language processing appear vulnerable. Regardless of the severity or type of injury, expressive language functions such as word fluency and naming problems are common (Ewing-Cobbs, Miner, Fletcher, & Levin, 1989). Problems in object description and naming have been observed even following mild brain injury (Ewing-Cobbs, Levin, Eisenberg, & Fletcher, 1987). Naming problems may continue to affect academic performance. Discourse problems also are commonly seen as the child recovers. They include issues with the use of syntactic rules that govern the formation of sentences so that length and complexity of verbal output is reduced (Hartley, 1995). Discourse-level language involves the successful integration of general knowledge, language comprehension, inferential skills, and other cognitive processes. Children with TBI, particularly those with severe injuries, can display persistent deficits in discourse-level language abilities long into the recovery process (Chapman et al., 1998).

Visuospatial Skills

Visuospatial skills are commonly impaired during the acute stages of recovery from TBI. Visuospatial skills involve visual perception abilities to scan, discriminate, analyze, recognize, and interpret what a person sees. They also involve construction skills that call upon the ability to create visual stimuli using perceptual skills and motor responses. In addition to difficulties involving higher-level visuospatial skills, children who have sustained a brain injury may have visual acuity impairments resulting from cranial nerve injuries, skull fractures, or brain swelling. Deficits of double vision, blurred vision, and decreased peripheral vision also are commonly reported and may affect the child's ability to process visual information and to read. Visual neglect for one side or one quadrant of the visual field is most commonly associated with right-hemisphere brain damage. Visual neglect can affect reading as well as practical activities such as dressing and grooming. Depending on the nature of the damage (permanent or transitory), visuospatial impairments may improve as the child recovers.

Executive Functions

Executive functioning involves the capacities for goal setting, self-direction, self-control, and self-regulation (Stuss, 1991). More specifically, executive functioning includes the ability to reason, problem solve, set goals, prioritize, self-monitor, self-correct, self-regulate, initiate or inhibit responses, organize and plan, and effectively execute purposeful behavior (Jantz & Coulter, 2007). Executive functioning impairments are associated most closely with prefrontal lobe injury (e.g., Levin et al., 1993; Levin et al., 1997), which often occurs as a result of trauma. When considering whether children with TBI have executive functioning impairments, it is important to control for maturational factors. This is because executive functioning is the slowest of all cognitive domains to develop completely. Nonetheless, children recovering from brain injury may have particular difficulty (relative to their peers) in setting goals, organizing behavior, monitoring and evaluating performance, shifting strategies in the event of failure, and remaining focused over time. These abilities are all important for success in "real world" academic environments. In addition, executive dysfunction may be demonstrated as social disinhibition, difficulty reading social cues, and impaired organization and monitoring of complex social responses. The demand for these social skills increases with a child's development and maturity (Slomine et al., 2002). Thus, problems in this area may become more apparent over time as expectations rise.

CONCLUSION

TBI in children typically results in a variety of neurocognitive and linguistic problems that can have a significant impact on the child's current status and future development. The PTBI was designed to assess the integrity of these critical skills during the recovery process and at various stages in the child's development. Chapter 3 provides information on the development of the PTBI.

3

Test Development

Prior to the development of the PTBI, no standardized test was available to assess specifically the neurocognitive and linguistic impairments associated with pediatric brain injury. The challenge we faced in designing the PTBI was to create a test that accounted for developmental and maturational changes as well as the neurocognitive and linguistic sequelae of brain injury.

In constructing the PTBI, the coauthors drew on their expertise in the areas of pediatric brain injury, child language development, and neuropsychology to develop a conceptual framework that would include cognitive and linguistic skills important to children who are developing typically as well as those skills most vulnerable to brain injury. During the initial phases of test development, potential subtests were proposed; of these, some were selected for piloting, and a pool of items was generated to conform to the construct, content, and format of each. Promising subtests and items were evaluated in a series of pilot studies involving more than 500 children. Based on the results of these pilot efforts, items and subtests were culled, and additional sets of items were generated. Some subtests were discarded, and others were modified and revised.

IRT methods, as well as classical test theory techniques, were used to establish item reliability and validity and to evaluate potential item-level bias. IRT analysis permits a scaling of item difficulty against the ability of the children tested. This made it possible to consider whether the range of difficulty for the set of items was appropriate for the ability range of the sample population. The additional application of differential item functioning methods made it possible to discard items that were biased for children belonging to different gender, cultural-linguistic, or racial/ethnic groups. Detailed information about these analyses can be found in Chapter 6. Finally, the conceptual model of the test was peer-reviewed prior to publication in the professional literature (Hotz et al., 2001; Hotz et al., 2009), and clinicians participating in the standardization research provided input about the test administration and scoring.

The standardization of the PTBI was conducted in two phases. Phase I (2007) involved completion of a small trial based on data collection from 44 children (32 children with TBI across the age range of 6–16 years as well as 12 typically developing children in the same age range). Protocols were collected from five different test sites that had Institutional Review Board (IRB) approval. These were evaluated and revised based on the IRT analyses.

Phase II began in January 2008 using a research version of the PTBI that was approved for administration by IRBs at 15 sites. Most of these sites (see Acknowledgments) were pediatric hospitals with programs for children with brain injuries who were in the acute care and rehabilitation phases of treatment. Feedback from the clinicians at these sites was used to make final adjustments to the Test Form, the directions to examiners, the scoring criteria, and the instructions to test takers. The regional distribution of children across several regions of the United States and Canada is evident in the Acknowledgments at the beginning of this manual.

Data were gathered for three groups of children ages 6–16 years:

1. Children who sustained a TBI
2. Children who sustained other forms of ABI (e.g., stroke, brain tumors, seizure disorders, encephalitis)
3. Children who were not affected by brain injury

No effort was made to exclude children with learning disabilities or developmental language disorders. These children, therefore, represent the typical, general population of children rather than a select population of "typical" children. The number and gender of children in each of these groups are described in Table 3.1. This final version of the PTBI has been administered to a total of 257 children, including 134 with TBI, 46 with ABI, and 77 who are typically developing. The gender and race/ethnicity classifications of participants in the sample are included in Tables 3.1 and 3.2.

Ten subtests had appropriate psychometric characteristics for inclusion in the PTBI. Three subtests assess developmentally constrained skills, which develop early and remain stable thereafter (see Chapter 4). They are as follows:

- Subtest 1: Orientation
- Subtest 2: Following Commands
- Subtest 6: Naming

Seven other subtests measure skills that are considered unconstrained, in that they show an extended period of development across the age span tested by the PTBI (see Chapter 4). They are as follows:

- Subtest 3: Word Fluency
- Subtest 4: What Goes Together

Table 3.1. Age and gender distributions of the 257 children used to establish item difficulty levels for the PTBI by diagnostic category

		Age (years)											
Category	Sex	6	7	8	9	10	11	12	13	14	15	16	Totals
TBI	Males	3	2	6	5	5	8	13	19	9	7	10	87
	Females	2	3	3	2	1	1	3	3	10	8	11	47
ABI	Males	3	0	2	2	1	2	2	2	2	7	0	23
	Females	3	1	4	0	2	2	2	2	1	4	2	23
Typical	Males	3	5	5	4	1	1	2	2	3	2	1	29
	Females	7	9	7	1	8	3	5	2	2	1	3	48
Total		21	20	27	14	18	17	27	30	27	29	27	257

Key: ABI, acquired brain injury. For the 46 participants with ABI, etiologies were reported as follows: 10 stroke, 6 anoxic, 5 intracerebral hemorrhage, 3 encephalitis, 7 brain tumor, 5 arteriovenous malformation, 2 metabolic, 3 seizure disorder, and 5 "other." *TBI*, traumatic brain injury. Of the 134 participants with TBI, 83 had initial scores reported for the Glasgow Coma Scale; of these, there were 42 severe, 7 moderate, and 34 mild.

Table 3.2. Demographic characteristics of the three subsamples of children

	TBI	ABI	Typical
Race/ethnicity			
African American	22	11	9
Asian	0	2	1
Hispanic (any race)	14	6	1
Native American	1	0	0
Caucasian	86	22	62
Other	9	3	4
Unreported	2	2	0
Languages spoken/understood			
English only	115	38	72
English and Spanish	11	5	2
English and other	7	3	0
Unreported	1	0	3
Languages read/written			
English only	120	41	71
English and Spanish	6	2	1
English and other	6	1	0
Spanish only	0	1	0
Unreported	2	1	5
Classroom performance			
Below average	15	9	0
Average	64	19	36
Above average	48	13	31
Unreported	7	5	10
Previous head injury			
Yes	117	1	0
No	12	42	67
Unreported	5	3	10
Premorbid handedness			
Right	115	40	67
Left	14	5	7
Ambidextrous	4	1	1
Unknown	1	0	2

Key: ABI, children with acquired brain injury; TBI, children with traumatic brain injury; Typical, typically developing children (no brain injury)

- Subtest 5: Digit Span
- Subtest 7: Story Retelling—Immediate
- Subtest 8: Yes/No/Maybe
- Subtest 9: Picture Recall
- Subtest 10: Story Retelling—Delayed

CONCLUSION

This chapter described the development and standardization of the PTBI on children 6–16 years old. The conceptual framework and rationale for the test are explored in Chapter 4.

4

Conceptual Framework and Rationale

CONCEPTUAL FRAMEWORK

The PTBI uses a conceptual framework of cognitive-linguistic abilities that are both developmentally appropriate for children and adolescents and particularly at risk following brain injury in this population. The "developmentally appropriate" principle led us to design measures for the PTBI using sentence- and discourse-level language reflecting higher-level processing expectations of the general education curriculum. The "particularly-at-risk" principle led us to design measures that would be sensitive to cognitive-linguistic processes that are likely to be affected by brain injury in early acute phases and more severe forms as well as later in recovery and in milder forms. An equally important principle was to keep the test brief enough to be usable in early acute phases but also broad enough to continue through later phases of rehabilitation, school reentry, and new learning. The theoretical and evidence-based model for the PTBI (i.e., based on factor analysis of results for the standardization research) appears in Figure 4.1 (see also Chapter 6).

This model represents a mix of skills that incorporate both higher-level and lower-level cognitive-linguistic processing skills in a 30-minute test. The constrained skills subtests reflect skills that are appropriate for measuring acute and severe problems but with limited developmental change across the school-age years. There is little variation in the scores from these subtests, reflecting their nature as constrained skills. The scores from the remaining subtests show noteworthy variability across individuals of different ages and diagnostic status, consistent with the notion that they measure unconstrained skills. These subtests are clustered in Figure 4.1 according to the statistical evidence that suggests performance on these subtests requires common underlying skills. The model is divided into five components:

- *Basic skills*—Basic skill (constrained) tasks capture evidence of confused orientation (Subtest 1: Orientation), difficulty following simple commands (Subtest 2: Following Commands), and anomia for common objects (Subtest 6: Naming).
- *Factor 1*—Factor 1 skills reflect unconstrained developmental language abilities for meeting curricular cognitive-linguistic demands, including language comprehension and inferential reasoning (Subtest 8: Yes/No/Maybe) and narration (Subtest 7: Story

<table>
<tr><td rowspan="4">Basic skills
(constrained developmental skills)

1. Orientation
2. Following Commands
6. Naming (anomia)</td><td colspan="3">Skills that develop across the school-age years
(unconstrained developmental skills)</td></tr>
<tr><td>Factor 1
Developmental language abilities for meeting curricular cognitive-linguistic demands
• Narration
• Discourse comprehension and inference</td><td>Factor 2
Complex cognitive-linguistic processes likely to be affected by brain injury
• Recall and organization of semantically related information
• Flexible thinking about relationships</td><td>Factor 3
Attention and immediate memory</td></tr>
<tr><td>7. Story Retelling—Immediate
8. Yes/No/Maybe
10. Story Retelling—Delayed</td><td>9. Picture Recall
4. What Goes Together</td><td>5. Digit Span</td></tr>
<tr><td colspan="3">Skills that reflect complex abilities
(related to Factors 1–3)
3. Word Fluency
4. What Goes Together (loads heavier on Factor 2, but also on Factors 1 and 3)</td></tr>
</table>

Figure 4.1. Evidence-based model showing conceptual framework for PTBI subtests.

Retelling—Immediate; Subtest 10: Story Retelling—Delayed). These are abilities that develop across the school-age years as contextual demands grow.

- *Factor 2*—Factor 2 skills reflect unconstrained complex cognitive-linguistic processes likely to be affected by brain injury, including visual-spatial perception, as well as mental manipulation and organization of graphic and semantic symbols (Subtest 9: Picture Recall; Subtest 4: What Goes Together). These abilities show developmental progression across the age range of the PTBI.
- *Factor 3*—Factor 3 skills reflect lower-level but unconstrained cognitive skills of attention and immediate memory (Subtest 5: Digit Span). These skills also show developmental growth across the age range of the PTBI.
- *Skills that reflect complex abilities*—All three factors operate somewhat equally for two of the subtests (Subtest 3: Word Fluency; Subtest 4: What Goes Together), showing the complex nature of word-level language processing tasks that require close attention, maintenance of cognitive set, and immediate and working memory.

CONCEPTS OF COMPLEXITY AND DIFFICULTY IN THE PTBI

As a new kind of evidence-based test, the PTBI and its subtests reflect concepts both of complexity and difficulty. *Complexity* is defined according to theory-based assumptions about what is likely to make a task difficult for those completing it; *difficulty* is defined operationally based on how well a task actually is performed by a particular group of people.

In developing the PTBI, we started with theoretical models of language and discourse complexity as well as with awareness of the cognitive-control processes that are likely to be compromised by brain injury in children and adolescents who were still developing and learning in school. The standardization data then were used to generate empirically derived ability scores that reflect the cumulative difficulty of items passed for use in the actual interpretation of results.

RATIONALE FOR THE PTBI SUBTESTS

The sections that follow offer further explanation of the theoretical rationale and cognitive-linguistic demands for each of the subtests. We emphasize that these subtests are designed for *assessment* of cognitive-linguistic sequelae of brain injury. They can point to areas to observe in further informal, contextualized (including curriculum-based), and dynamic assessment activities. The assessment tasks should not be used to provide stimuli for treatment, nor should they be used as models of what to do in treatment.

Subtest 1: Orientation

Establishing status of orientation is particularly important early in the recovery process. Orientation requires memory for old and new information and language skills for understanding and answering questions. Difficulties may reflect disorientation, confusion, or memory or language problems. A finding of low performance on this subtest provides important information about a child's status, but a finding of high performance does not by itself mean that the child is asymptomatic of brain injury.

Subtest 2: Following Commands

The ability to follow commands accurately is important for participating in home and school activities as well as in rehabilitation programs. The Following Commands subtest requires children to attend, understand the language of spoken commands, and retain the essence of each component while organizing and executing an accurate gestural response. Difficulty with following commands is not a simple function of adding steps. Even though young children can follow most simple commands without difficulty before they enter school, this apparently simple ability requires integration and representation of linguistically encoded information using perceptual-motor processes that cross domains. Commands with complex syntax are those that require a sequence of responding that does not correspond to the order of mention in the sentence. Items with complex syntax include, "*Before* you point to the floor, point to your foot" and, "Point to the light *after* you shake your head." Both of these items require the child to perform the actions in a sequence different from the order mentioned in the sentence.

Subtest 3: Word Fluency

The Word Fluency subtest calls on multiple skills for conducting an organized search of the mental lexicon, first by semantic category and then by initial letter. It also requires working memory for holding previously mentioned responses in memory so as not to repeat them. The timed nature (1 minute each for semantic and phonemic tasks) puts added pressure on children with slowed mental processing skills. The results of this subtest provide information about performance difficulty a child or adolescent with brain injury might have when attempting a complex cognitive-linguistic, word-level task.

Subtest 4: What Goes Together

The What Goes Together subtest taps semantic/conceptual knowledge, categorical awareness, and mental flexibility. Semantic/conceptual knowledge provides the building blocks for language acquisition and use. In the school-age years, vocabulary knowledge incorporates awareness of semantic hierarchies and of categorical as well as functional relationships. The What Goes Together subtest also requires examinees to formulate a spoken response, drawing on integrated cognitive-linguistic skills and retrieval of words and phrases for expressing core relationships. This verbalization requirement increases the complexity of the task demands.

Subtest 5: Digit Span

The Digit Span subtest is primarily a test of attention and immediate memory. Digit Span performance may be low in the acute phases of brain injury but then recover independent of tasks with higher-level cognitive demands (Lezak et al., 2004). Although Digit Span is a relatively low-level task, data for the PTBI standardization showed it to develop across the school-age span of the test. Processing, storing, and verbalizing numbers depends on an intact language system. The presence of aphasia, as well as attention and memory deficits, may lead to poor performance on this task.

Subtest 6: Naming

Naming parts of a picture requires visual-perceptual as well as word retrieval skills. Decontextualized naming, in which a child is requested to name objects pointed to by an examiner, also is called *confrontation naming*. Naming deficits are a key symptom of both aphasia and diffuse brain damage. Slightly delayed retrieval may be a sign of mild anomia. It is important to note, however, that naming difficulties can be relatively unpredictable and difficult to measure in their milder forms. Even if a child shows high or moderate performance on this task, he or she may show word-finding difficulties in naturalistic contexts.

Subtest 7: Story Retelling—Immediate

Three grade-appropriate stories were constructed with classic story grammar structure (setting, initiating event/problem, internal response, attempt, outcome, ending) (Stein & Glenn, 1982). The stories reflect age-appropriate themes at different grade levels. Inferential relationships and figurative language are embedded in the stories. The Story Retelling subtest calls on highly integrated and sophisticated cognitive-linguistic skills, including language comprehension, higher-level discourse ability, memory, and language reformulation. Children who are able to use a discourse macrostructure framework should be able to remember more parts of the story. Story retelling also permits examiners to observe children's abilities to form grammatically correct, complete sentences.

Subtest 8: Yes/No/Maybe

Comprehension of varied types of syntactic and discourse structures are an essential ability for performing well in school. The Yes/No/Maybe subtest is made up of short "stories," which were constructed using curriculum discourse as the model with an emphasis on complex syntax. The printed stories remain available to the children, which reduces the working memory load and makes it possible for students with reading skills and strategies associated with executive functions to perform better. The primary purpose of the subtest is to assess language comprehension. This subtest requires higher-level language comprehension skills supported by sophisticated information processing skills, including attention, mental tracking, and evaluation of possible responses.

Subtest 9: Picture Recall

Visual memory problems can present major barriers to academic and everyday functioning. The Picture Recall subtest assesses incidental memory for the picture presented in an earlier subtest. Incidental memory is a form of memory wherein the individual is not alerted in advance to the possible need to recall a set of information at a later time.

Subtest 10: Story Retelling—Delayed

Delayed discourse recall is critical for all aspects of academic functioning. Teachers typically discuss information during more than 1 day in class, making it essential to remember discourse over an extended amount of time. The Story Retelling—Delayed subtest requires long-term memory as well as highly integrated and sophisticated cognitive-linguistic skills, including language comprehension, higher-level discourse ability, memory, and language reformulation. Children with brain injury typically have encoding difficulties, making retrieval of information after a short time delay particularly problematic.

CONCLUSION

The PTBI uses a conceptual framework of cognitive-linguistic abilities that are 1) developmentally appropriate for children and adolescents and 2) particularly at risk following brain injury. The concepts of complexity and difficulty are reflected in the subtests. Chapter 5 provides administration and scoring directions for the PTBI.

5

Administration and Scoring Directions

EXAMINERS' RESPONSIBILITIES

Examiners administering the PTBI should have training and experience in administering and interpreting individualized assessments of children and adolescents. Before beginning, it is essential to read all PTBI instructions and administration procedures. You should be prepared to conduct testing without stopping to familiarize yourself with administration procedures and, thereby, interrupting the flow of testing. Follow procedures carefully. Failure to do so may invalidate test results. Keep the following points in mind while administering the test:

- Do not test individuals who are agitated or upset.
- Discontinue testing if an individual becomes agitated or upset during testing.
- Do not discuss PTBI performance with examinees during administration. If examinees ask how they are doing, say, "You're doing fine. We can talk about that more after we're finished."
- Do not tell examinees whether their responses were correct or incorrect.
- Do not provide leading questions, prompts, or probes that may serve as cues. If examinees do not understand the task requirements of a certain subtest, even with the designated instructions (i.e., are not in task "set"), discontinue the subtest. In such cases, indicate on the score form that the subtest could not be administered, and do not assign any score.
- Do not use the PTBI tasks for practice or treatment under any circumstances.
- Protect the PTBI test materials and results. PTBI results are part of an individual's medical records and, therefore, are confidential. Results should be discussed only with those with the legal right to know. Test protocols and/or materials should not be given to family members and other nontrained people. Reports of test results should be made available only to those authorized by the patient or his or her legal guardian with the legal rights to do so.

GENERAL INFORMATION

A standardized test is administered in a "standard" manner. *Do not vary* from the PTBI administration procedures as they are written in the PTBI Test Form. Use the following guidelines throughout testing:

- Administer all PTBI subtests in the order they appear in the Test Form, beginning with Subtest 1 (Orientation) and ending with Subtest 10 (Story Retelling—Delayed).
- Administer the PTBI in two sessions if examinees have limited capacity for test taking or if administration time is limited. In such cases, the PTBI *must be given in two sessions within the same day.* All the memory tasks are included in the latter portion (Subtests 6–10) of the PTBI; therefore, when administering the PTBI in two sessions, end the first session after Subtest 5 (Digit Span) and begin the second session with Subtest 6 (Naming).
- Follow all specific directions for administering the PTBI subtests and for recording and scoring examinees' responses.
- Read the key instructions printed in the instruction banners at the top of each subtest in the PTBI Test Form.

TESTING ENVIRONMENT

Take the following steps to establish a testing environment that promotes optimal performance from each examinee:

- Schedule and administer the PTBI at a time when the examinee is most likely to be alert and rested.
- Administer the test in the most quiet, least distracting environment possible.
- Position the examinee so it is not possible to see a calendar or other environmental prompts (e.g., pictures of animals).
- Position the Test Form so that the examinee cannot read the scores.
- Sit directly across from the examinee or, if at the examinee's bedside, at a comfortable angle.
- Use a flat surface cleared of distracting stimuli when displaying visual materials and for the drawing/writing task (Subtest 9: Picture Recall).

TEST SUPPLIES

Examiners will need the following materials each time the PTBI is administered:

- PTBI Test Form
- PTBI Stimulus Book
- Black ink pen, preferably fine point and felt-tipped

- Timepiece for recording time in seconds
- Calculator

PROMPTS AND PROBES

Keep in mind the following definitions of *prompts* and *probes* as you administer the PTBI:

- A *prompt* is a neutral form of encouragement (e.g., "You can keep going," "We have to move along," "You have time to check your work"). During testing, use only neutral prompts such as "We're moving along" or "Only a few more."
- A *probe* is a cue for more specific information; only those probes described in the PTBI Test Form may be used.

REPEATING DIRECTIONS AND STIMULI

Permitted repetitions are stated in the instruction banner for each subtest in the Test Form.

- A single repetition of a task instruction or item is used only when examinees:

  Appear not to understand task instructions or items

  Request a repetition of instructions or items

  Do not respond within 10 seconds
- Indicate on the Test Form when repetitions are used.
- If examinees fail to respond after one repetition and have still not responded for 10 seconds, note *NR* for *no response* and proceed to the next item or subtest.

TIME LIMITS

Note the following about time limits for the PTBI:

- The average administration time for the PTBI is 30 minutes.
- Only one subtest (Subtest 3: Word Fluency) has set time limits.
- All subtests require examinees to begin responding within 10 seconds of introduction of the items; after 10 seconds, the instruction or stimulus item can be repeated one time.
- If no response is forthcoming within 10 seconds after the repetition, the next item is introduced.
- The total time for standard administration of the PTBI should not exceed 45 minutes.
- You, as the examiner, should control the testing session so that examinees inclined toward tangential or excessive responding do not do so. In such cases, use neutral prompts, such as "We must keep going" or "You can tell me about that later" to keep testing on track.

- Space has been provided to record *administration time* for subtests. You are encouraged to note times because notable changes in response time upon retesting(s) can provide a way to measure recovery (shorter response times are positive signs of recovery) or newly occurring problems (longer response times may be indicative of new problems).

It is important to note that some subtests have rules for discontinuation that appear in the instruction banner printed on the Test Form. These rules must be followed for standardized testing.

RECORDING RESPONSES

Please make note of the following guidelines for recording responses to questions on the PTBI.

- On the PTBI Test Form, space is provided for you to record examinees' exact responses to most subtests. You are strongly encouraged to write the exact responses of examinees for qualitative review of performance characteristics.
- The notes for examiners at the end of each subtest offer suggestions for qualitative review of incorrect responses. Qualitative reviews of error responses may lead to better understanding of the nature of the individual's difficulties.
- Directions and values for quantitative scoring of responses to each subtest are clearly indicated on the Test Form.

OBTAINING PTBI CRITERION SCORES

Criterion scores are used to compare an individual's performance to a standard for judging the adequacy of skill performance. The PTBI permits the calculation of an ability score to describe current skill level for each subtest; it provides four performance categories that describe ranges of ability scores for each subtest. These categories include Very Low, Low, Moderate, and High performance. Finally, the PTBI provides a standard error of measurement (*SEM*) for computing a confidence interval to assist in determining when changes in scores represent true changes in ability when the test is re-administered over time.

How to Obtain Ability Scores

Ability scores provide a numerical index of a child's current ability to respond to subtest items of different difficulty levels. Ability scores can be used to establish current skill levels and to track change over time.

It is critical that the PTBI be administered exactly as the directions prescribe and be scored consistent with the examples in the Examiner's Manual in order for the ability scores to apply. Any deviation from the standard procedures for administration and scoring can cause significant changes in the difficulty level of the test as administered. This will cause incorrect interpretations of current ability levels and prevent the ability to track change with time. Significant deviations from standard administration (e.g., providing help with answering items) also may invalidate the test for future use.

Follow these instructions to obtain an ability score:

- For Subtest 3: Word Fluency, simply add the total number of words produced.
- For the remaining subtests, ability scores are used. Follow these instructions:

  Notice that the Test Form includes an ability score rather than the traditional 0 or 1 scoring.

  As you score the test, cross out the item ability scores for each of the items missed. Circle the ability scores for correct items.

  To obtain a total ability score for each subtest, add the circled ability scores (i.e., for items passed) on the subtest.

  The total ability scores possible are provided on the Test Form.

  The total number of points possible reflects both the difficulty of the items within the subtest AND the number of items within a subtest. Therefore, ability levels are not intended to be compared across subtests. Always consider the ability score relative to the total possible score within that subtest.

Scoring and Summarizing PTBI Performance

This section describes the procedures for summarizing item ability scores and verifying earned scores:

1. Total the correct (circled) responses for each subtest. This will allow you to compute the total ability scores for each subtest.

   Example: For Subtest 1: Orientation, the highest possible total ability score is 38.0. For example, if the child responds correctly to items 1, 2, 3a, 3b, 3c, 4, 5, 10, and 11, he or she would receive an ability total score of 22.5 on this subtest. This is the total ability score for Subtest 1, and this number will be recorded in the Ability Score column of the Summary Scoring Chart on page 1 of the Test Form.

2. Match the ability score to a performance category of High, Moderate, Low, or Very Low using the table in Appendix A that corresponds to the child's age.

   Example: For the 8-year-old child with an ability score of 22.5 on Subtest 1: Orientation, the child's performance would fall in the Low performance category. Place a checkmark in the box for Low in the Performance Category column in the Summary Scoring Chart on page 1 of the Test Form.

3. Find the *SEM* values for each subtest using the table column in Appendix B that corresponds to the child's age. Enter the values on the Scoring Summary Chart in the *SEM* column. These values will be used to compute the confidence intervals and judge the significance of any changes in scores for a child who was tested previously.

   Example: For an 8-year-old child who receives a score of 22.5 on Subtest 1: Orientation, the table in Appendix B indicates an *SEM* of 2 for the Orientation subtest at age 8.

4. Subtract the *SEM* from the subtest total ability score to find the lower confidence interval value. (*Note:* The lowest possible value is 0.) Add the *SEM* to the subtest total

ability score to find the upper confidence interval value. Enter these values in the Summary Scoring Chart on page 1 of the Test Form in the column labeled Confidence Interval.

Example: For a score of 22.5 and a confidence interval value of 2, the lower confidence interval value would be 20.5, and the upper confidence interval value would be 24.5. This is the score range that a child would have to exceed to demonstrate true improvement (or regression) rather than random variability on any subsequent testing with the PTBI. The confidence interval would be recorded on the Test Form as "20.5 to 24.5."

5. After scoring all subtests, you will be able to report a performance profile pattern for the child by looking at the levels of performance on each subtest.

   Example: For the 8-year-old child, you might report a performance pattern of mostly Low across subtests if that is what is indicated. Or, you might find and report an overall performance pattern of Low to Moderate. Other children may be highly variable in their performance, with performance categories ranging from Very Low to High.

6. If the child has been tested previously with the PTBI, enter the date in the Previous Test Results column. Record the total ability score and performance category ratings earned at that time. These can be compared with the child's current ability score and current performance category to gauge whether change is significant by considering whether the prior and current confidence intervals overlap. (If they do not, the change is significant.)

   Example: The 8-year-old child in this example previously responded correctly to Items 1, 2, 3c, 4, and 5 on the Orientation subtest, earning a total ability score of 10.5, which fell in the Very Low range (see Figure 5.1). The upper confidence interval from the previous test (not included on the current Summary Scoring Chart) was 12.5. Thus, the child's retest score on the Orientation subtest, which is now in the confidence interval 20.5 to 24.5, has increased significantly from the previous test, moving from the Very Low to the Low performance category.

Please note that the performance rating on each subtest and the overall performance summary on the PTBI are appropriate to report for medical and school records (see Chapter 7 for sample reports).

SUMMARY SCORING CHART	Ability Score (from Test Form)	Performance Category (from Appendix A)	*SEM*	Confidence Interval	Previous Test Results
Constrained Skills		**VL** = Very Low **L** = Low **M** = Moderate **H** = High	Standard error of measurement (from Appendix B)	Add and subtract *SEM* from Ability Score	Date: 3 months prior Ability Score Perf. Category
1. Orientation	22.5	☐ VL ☑ L ☐ M ☐ H	2	20.5 to 24.5	10.5 VL

Figure 5.1. Summary Scoring Chart indicating previous test results for an 8-year-old child.

ADMINISTERING AND SCORING INDIVIDUAL PTBI SUBTESTS

Unambiguous procedures have been established for administering and scoring individual PTBI subtests. These procedures are described in the Test Form and are as follows:

- An instruction banner is displayed on the Test Form at the top of each PTBI subtest. This banner provides information about the test materials, instructions, discontinue and repetition rules, and scoring.

- A behavioral observations checklist for tracking and noting such behaviors as attention, responsiveness, and perseveration appears at the bottom of each subtest, along with space to record other behaviors:

  Use the checklists to make observations about examinees' responses and behaviors, such as requests for repetitions, delayed responding, perseverations, unintelligible responses, failure to produce any response (no response), and self-corrections.

  Verbal responses also can be analyzed for paraphasic errors such as those produced by individuals with aphasia or confused language.

  Extra space is provided for recording any unusual or inappropriate behavior displayed by examinees (e.g., signs of anger, frustration, agitation, social inappropriateness). Decreases in these behaviors across repeated administration of the PTBI can be indicative of natural recovery and/or positive response to treatment. Increases in these behaviors upon follow-up testing may be "red flags" for new neurologic conditions (e.g., seizure activity), psychological reactions (e.g., depression), pain, or other types of problems.
- Notes for examiners also appear at the bottom of each subtest. These notes provide information about behaviors to observe during test administration and possible interpretations and conclusions to be drawn from examinees' performance on each subtest.

Subtest 1: Orientation

During this subtest, examinees respond verbally to 11 questions probing orientation to person, place, and date.

Special Instructions

- Repeat each question one time if examinees appear not to understand the question, if they ask for a repetition, or if they fail to respond within 10 seconds.
- If examinees give an incomplete response to multipart question number 3 ("When is your birthday?"), probe for each component of the response.

Recording and Scoring Subtest Responses

- Record all spoken responses verbatim, and note any unusual nonverbal behaviors. Credit only verbal responses.
- Do not allow written responses, except where indicated in the Test Form.
- Do not allow use of communication books, calendars, or other compensatory memory devices.
- Score each answer according to the point values listed for each item. These point values were established by IRT procedures (see Chapter 6). The item point values appear in the right-hand column.
- Add all earned scores to calculate the Total Orientation Ability Score.
- Record time to administer.

See Figure 5.2 for an example of scoring of the Orientation subtest.

Item	Question/Response	Ability Score
1	***What is your full name?*** (Child must say both first and last name. If child does not say last name on first trial, **probe** for last name.)	(0.5)
2	***How old are you?*** 16 (DR)	(1.5)
3a	***When is your birthday?*** (For incomplete responses, **probe** for month, day, and year.) Month December	~~2.0~~
3b	Day 17th	~~2.0~~
3c	Year IDK	~~3.5~~
4	***What grade are you in?*** 10th (DR) (If summer, accept either completed or upcoming grade.)	(2.0)
5	***What school do you go to?*** Kennedy High School (DR)	(3.0)
6	***What city or town do you live in?*** (NR) (If rural address, accept nearest town.)	~~4.0~~
7	***What state/province do you live in?*** 17th (P)	~~3.5~~
8	***What is this place?*** IDK (Accept "hospital," "clinic," "school," "home," and so forth.)	~~3.5~~
9	***What day of the week is it today?*** IDK	~~4.5~~
10	***What month is it?*** IDK	~~4.0~~
11	***What year is it?*** IDK	~~4.0~~

Time to administer: 4 min. **TOTAL ORIENTATION ABILITY SCORE** 7.0 / 38.0

Behavioral observations: (Abbreviations may be used next to items where they apply.)

___ Repetition of instructions (Rep)	✓ Perseveration (P)	✓ No response (NR)
___ Attention reminder required (Attn)	✓ Delayed response (5+ sec) (DR)	✓ I don't know (IDK)
___ Prompt to reestablish set (Prompt)	___ Unintelligible response (UnR)	___ Self-correction (SC)

Additional qualitative/behavioral observations:

Slow responder

Disoriented to time and place

Figure 5.2. Subtest 1: Orientation. *Examinee:* 16-year-old male in 10th grade tested 1-week post closed head injury—all terrain vehicle, small anterior interhemispheric falx hemorrhage. (*Note:* The birth month and day given were incorrect.)

Subtest 2: Following Commands

During this subtest, examinees respond nonverbally to spoken commands that have been ordered according to difficulty as established by IRT procedures.

Special Instructions

- Repeat each command one time if examinees ask for a repetition or fail to respond within 10 seconds.
- Discourage verbalizations during execution of the actions.

Recording and Scoring Subtest Responses

- Record all motor/gestural responses, and note any unusual verbal behaviors.
- Score motor/gestural responses only according to the scoring criteria as determined by IRT procedures for establishing difficulty levels.

- Add all earned item scores for Total Following Commands Ability Score.
- Record time to administer.

See Figure 5.3 for an example of scoring of the Following Commands subtest.

Subtest 3: Word Fluency

This subtest consists of two tasks. In the first task, examinees verbally list as many animals as possible in 1 minute. In the second task, examinees list as many words beginning with the letter *M* as possible in 1 minute.

Special Instructions

- Be prepared to time this subtest using a timepiece with a seconds hand.
- The recording section of the Test Form is arranged in four columns to enable you to capture responses in 15-second intervals.
- For the semantic fluency category (animal naming), show examinees the word *ANIMALS* on page 1 of the Stimulus Book.
- For the phonemic fluency task (*M* words), show examinees the letter *M* on page 2 of the Stimulus Book.
- Repeat each command one time if examinees ask for a repetition or fail to respond within 10 seconds. If examinees stop listing items before 1 minute is up, say, "Keep going. You have time left." This prompt can be given only once.

Item	Command/Response	Ability Score
1	***Where's your knee?***	(0.5)
2	***Make a fist.***	(1.5)
3	***Stick out your tongue and then point to the door.***	(1.5)
4	***Before you point to the floor, point to your foot.***	(1.5)
5	***After you look at the ceiling, touch your heart.*** (DR) looked at ceiling while touching heart	~~1.5~~
6	***With your thumb, touch your stomach.***	(2.5)
7	***Look to the left and then to the right.***	(3.0)
8	***Point to the light after you shake your head.*** (DR) pointed to light while shaking head	~~3.0~~
Time to administer: 4 min.	**TOTAL FOLLOWING COMMANDS ABILITY SCORE**	10.5 / 15.0

Behavioral observations: (Abbreviations may be used next to items where they apply.)

__ Repetition of instructions (Rep)	__ Perseveration (P)	__ No response (NR)
__ Attention reminder required (Attn)	✓ Delayed response (5+ sec) (DR)	__ I don't know (IDK)
__ Prompt to reestablish set (Prompt)	__ Unintelligible response (UnR)	__ Self-correction (SC)

Additional qualitative/behavioral observations:

Appears not to be processing the relational term, "after."

Figure 5.3. Subtest 2: Following Commands. *Examinee*: ninth-grade male tested 6-weeks post traumatic brain injury—pedestrian hit by automobile, bifrontal and left temporal subarachnoid hemorrhage.

Recording and Scoring Subtest Responses

- Record examinees' responses verbatim in each of the 15-second increment columns provided in the Test Form for the semantic (animal naming) and phonemic (*M* words) categories.

For the semantic fluency (animal naming) task, follow these instructions:

- Identify correct, nonredundant responses that name any animal or category of animal, including exemplars of mammals, insects, birds, dinosaurs, fish, and so forth.
- Allow for mild dysarthria or slight mispronunciations, such as paraphasias in which the target is clearly identifiable (e.g., "crocopile").
- Do NOT count as correct the following:

  Any word that does not represent the animal kingdom (e.g., "plant")

  Perseverations (repetition of a previously correct response)

  Description of animals (e.g., "the one with the trunk")

  Names that do not represent different types of animals (e.g., "little bear" and "big bear" would be counted as one animal, as opposed to "black bear" and "brown bear," which *are* different types of bears and would count as two animals)

  Plurals of previously named animals (e.g., "dogs" after "dog")

  Diminutives of previously named animals (e.g., "horsey" after "horse")

  Nonwords (e.g., "wokies")

  Unintelligible responses

For the phonemic fluency (*M* word) task, follow these instructions:

- Identify correct, nonredundant responses that are real words beginning with the letter *M*.
- Allow for mild dysarthria or slight mispronunciations (e.g., accent on wrong syllable) in which the target is clearly identifiable.
- Do NOT count as correct the following:

  Any word that does not being with *M*

  Any word that is an inflection of another word that already has been named (e.g., "mother" after "mothers", "making" after "make"); however, words that are new derivations of the same base form do count separately (e.g., "mom" and "mother" would count as two words)

  Perseverations (repetition of a previously correct response)

  Nonwords (e.g., "maffer")

  Unintelligible responses

Add all the words that met the criteria for one point credit for the semantic and phonemic fluency categories for the Total Word Fluency Ability Score. See Figure 5.4 for an example of scoring of the Word Fluency subtest.

3A. Semantic: Animals

0–15 seconds	16–30 seconds	31–45 seconds	45–60 seconds
dog horse bird fish	cat chicken	"I can't think of any more"	

Animal Fluency Score 6

3B. Phonemic: *M* words

0–15 seconds	16–30 seconds	31–45 seconds	45–60 seconds
monkey mother Mom	"I can't think of any more"		

***M* Fluency Score** 3
Animal Fluency Score 6
TOTAL WORD FLUENCY SCORE 9

Behavioral observations: (Abbreviations may be used next to items where they apply.)

___ Repetition of instructions (Rep)	___ Perseveration (P)	___ No response (NR)
___ Attention reminder required (Attn)	___ Delayed response (5+ sec) (DR)	___ I don't know (IDK)
___ Prompt to reestablish set (Prompt)	___ Unintelligible response (UnR)	___ Self-correction (SC)

Additional qualitative/behavioral observations:

No error response but quickly runs out of steam and cannot sustain search

Figure 5.4. Subtest 3: Word Fluency. *Examinee*: 8-year, 6-month-old female in third grade tested 10 days post-fall—all terrain vehicle (unhelmeted), small right parietal subarachnoid hemorrhage, right orbital fracture, subarachnoid hemorrhage interpeduncular fossa.

Subtest 4: What Goes Together

During this subtest, examinees look at sets of three words displayed in the Stimulus Book (pp. 3–10) while the examiner reads the words aloud. Examinees are obliged to complete four operations for each set of three words: 1) indicate which two of three words go together, and 2) explain why they go together. After doing this for the first paired combination, examinees must 3) pair two different words, and 4) provide reasons for why they go together in a different way.

Special Instructions

- If examinees do not understand the nature of the task (i.e., cannot get into task "set"), even with practice on the practice item, then discontinue this subtest.
- Rules for repetitions are stated in instruction banners for each subtest. Comply with these rules.
- Do not ask examinees to read words aloud, but do not discourage them if they do.
- Examinees can either point to or say the word pairings.

- The order of the pairings does not matter.
- If examinees are unable to speak, provide paper and pen for them to write reasons for pairings. Staple their written response to the Test Form.

Recording and Scoring Subtest Responses

- Acceptable word pairs are printed in boldface. Examiners may circle word pairs to more easily identify correct and incorrect pairings for scoring.
- Always ask, "Why?" after each pairing response, even if the pairing is incorrect (e.g., *blue* and *apple*). Record all responses to facilitate qualitative analysis as well as for assigning ability scores if the pairings are correct and the "Why?" responses are acceptable. Acceptable responses for earning credit are listed on the Test Form under "Why?" (*Note:* Examiners may choose to simply circle the examinee's correct response if it matches what is listed in the Test Form.)
- Record all verbal responses verbatim in the space provided for each word pair. In order to receive credit for pairing, both word pairs must be correct (e.g., for *red, apple, blue,* examinees must pair *red* and *blue* and *red* and *apple*—in either order).
- Again, to receive credit for responses to "Why?" examinees must provide acceptable answers for acceptable pairs. No other responses earn credit.
- The credit values (as determined by IRT procedures) for each correct response to "Why?" are indicated on the Test Form (e.g., for *red* and *blue*, the only acceptable answer is *"They're both colors."* This response is worth 6.0; for *red* and *apple*, the only acceptable responses are "*Apple is red/can be red*" for 6.0).
- Add earned item scores for Total What Goes Together Ability Score.
- Record time to administer.

See Figure 5.5 for an example of scoring of the What Goes Together subtest.

Subtest 5: Digit Span

This subtest requires examinees to repeat series of numbers ranging from two numbers to seven numbers that are spoken aloud by the examiner. For each level of numbers, two exemplars are presented. Testing continues as long as at least one of the two items at a level is repeated correctly.

Special Instructions

- Read aloud the numbers at the rate of one number per second with equal and even stress and prosody.
- At least one of the two sets of numbers at each level must be repeated correctly to advance to the next level.

Item	Item Content/Responses	Ability Score	Item	Item Content/Responses	Ability Score
1a	red – apple – blue		1c	red – apple – blue	0.5
1b	**Why?** Make purple both colors	~~6.0~~	1d	**Why?** Both red apple is / can be red	~~6.0~~
2a	knife – fork – saw		2c	knife – fork – saw	5.0
2b	**Why?** Spikes things you eat with, utensils, silverware	~~2.5~~	2d	**Why?** both sharp, used to cut	3.5
3a	car – water – boat		3c	car – water – boat	6.0
3b	**Why?** Put people on both transportation, take you places, go in them / drive them, have motors	~~5.0~~	3d	**Why?** Boat goes on water boat goes in / moves in / across water	6.0
4a	mother – father – daughter		4c	mother – father – daughter	5.0
4b	**Why?** Like each other married, parents, takes two to make a daughter	~~4.5~~	4d	**Why?** females, girls, women, daughter comes from mother	2.5

Item	Item Content/Responses	Ability Score	Item	Item Content/Responses	Ability Score
5a	taste – nose – smell		5c	taste – nose – smell	6.0
5b	**Why?** IDK both senses (**not**—you can smell and taste food)	~~4.0~~	5d	**Why?** smell with nose, use nose to smell	1.5
6a	painter – elevator – ladder		6c	painter – elevator – ladder	5.0
6b	**Why?** Go up use to go up and down / reach high places (**not**—go up only)	~~5.0~~	6d	**Why?** painter uses / stands on ladder	5.5
7a	bat – eagle – owl		7c	bat – eagle – owl	6.0
7b	**Why?** both birds, have feathers	7.5	7d	**Why?** IDK nocturnal, up at night	~~7.5~~

Time to administer: 5 min. **Subtotal Score 1** 7.5 / 34.5

Subtotal Score 2 52.5 / 66.0
Subtotal Score 1 7.5 / 34.5
TOTAL WHAT GOES TOGETHER ABILTY SCORE 60.0 / 100.5

Behavioral observations: (Abbreviations may be used next to items where they apply.)

___ Repetition of instructions (Rep)	___ Perseveration (P)	___ No response (NR)
___ Attention reminder required (Attn)	✓ Delayed response (5+ sec) (DR)	✓ I don't know (IDK)
___ Prompt to reestablish set (Prompt)	___ Unintelligible response (UnR)	___ Self-correction (SC)

Additional qualitative/behavioral observations:
Often slow in responding

Figure 5.5. Subtest 4: What Goes Together. *Examinee*: 8-year, 2-month-old male in third grade tested 6 weeks post being struck on the head by a blunt instrument. Computed tomography (CT) showed cerebral edema.

Recording and Scoring Subtest Responses

- Record the numbers as spoken by examinees.
- To receive credit, examinees must repeat target numbers in the order given.
- Assign points as indicated in the right-hand column for each set of stimuli correctly repeated. These points were determined by IRT procedures.
- Discontinue the task if both sequences of numbers are incorrect at any level.
- Add earned item scores for Total Digit Span Ability Score.
- Record time to administer.

See Figure 5.6 for an example of scoring of the Digit Span subtest.

Item	Stimuli/Responses	Ability Score	Item	Stimuli/Responses	Ability Score
1a	***7 – 3***	(0.5)	1b	***5 – 9***	(0.5)
2a	***5 – 8 – 2***	(0.5)	2b	***4 – 1 – 8***	(1.0)
3a	***6 – 4 – 9 – 3***	(4.0)	3b	***8 – 2 – 5 – 1***	(5.0)
4a	***7 – 5 – 1 – 4 – 9*** 7 - 4	~~9.5~~	4b	***3 – 8 – 1 – 7 – 2*** 3 - 8 - 7 - 8 - 1 - 2	~~10.0~~
5a	***9 – 2 – 5 – 8 – 1 – 4***	~~11.5~~	5b	***2 – 5 – 9 – 6 – 3 – 8***	~~12.5~~
6a	***1 – 7 – 3 – 8 – 6 – 2 – 9***	~~13.5~~	6b	***7 – 2 – 5 – 8 – 1 – 9 – 4***	~~14.0~~

Time to administer: 3 min. **Subtotal Score 1** 5.0 / 39.5

Subtotal Score 2 6.5 / 43.0
Subtotal Score 1 5.0 / 39.5
TOTAL DIGIT SPAN ABILITY SCORE 11.5 / 82.5

Behavioral observations: (Abbreviations may be used next to items where they apply.)

___ Repetition of instructions (Rep)	✓ Perseveration (P)	___ No response (NR)
___ Attention reminder required (Attn)	___ Delayed response (5+ sec) (DR)	___ I don't know (IDK)
___ Prompt to reestablish set (Prompt)	___ Unintelligible response (UnR)	___ Self-correction (SC)

Additional qualitative/behavioral observations:

Perseverates on "8" item 4b

Figure 5.6. Subtest 5: Digit Span. *Examinee:* 8-year, 11-month-old female in second grade tested 5 months post fall from a moving car—multiple skull fractures, frontal/parietal epidural hematoma, diffuse axonal injury, craniotomy right frontal/parietal region.

Subtest 6: Naming

This subtest requires examinees to name body parts and objects as depicted in the "skateboarder" picture on page 11 of the Stimulus Book. (*Note:* If administering PTBI in two sessions, begin second session here.)

Special Instructions

- If writing is required, provide pen and paper and staple responses to the Test Form. Do not offer examinee a pencil with an eraser.
- If examinees do not see the target body part or object to be named, point more precisely and say, "No, this part/thing."
- Do NOT tell examinees to remember this picture.
- If examinees comment that the boy should be wearing a helmet, say, "You're exactly right. He should be wearing a helmet."

Recording and Scoring Subtest Responses

- Circle naming responses that are correct responses.
- Record incorrect naming responses verbatim as spoken by examinees.

Item	Question	Target Item/Response	Ability Score
1	***What do you call these things?*** (If child names "trucks," [part of a skateboard], say, ***"No, this part,"*** and point again, specifically to wheels)	(Wheels)	(0.5)
2	***What do you call these things?*** (If child names "laces" [or other part], say, ***"No, the whole thing."***)	Boots / (Shoes)	(0.5)
3	***What do you call this thing?***	(Star)	(0.5)
4	***What do you call this thing?***	Chain / ID tags / Dog tags / Necklace Put it around your neck; get one for Valentine's day	~~1.5~~
5	***What do you call this thing?***	Band-Aid Put it on a cut	~~2.0~~
6	***What do you call this part of his body?***	(Chin)	(2.0)
7	***And this part of his body?***	(Elbow) Arm elbow (SC)	(2.5)
8	***And this part?*** (If child names "eye" [or other part], say, ***"No, this part."***)	Eyebrow Eyelash	~~3.0~~

Time to administer: 3 min. **TOTAL NAMING ABILITY SCORE** 6.0 / 12.5

Behavioral observations: (Abbreviations may be used next to items where they apply.)

___ Repetition of instructions (Rep)	___ Perseveration (P)	___ No response (NR)
___ Attention reminder required (Attn)	___ Delayed response (5+ sec) (DR)	___ I don't know (IDK)
___ Prompt to reestablish set (Prompt)	___ Unintelligible response (UnR)	✓ Self-correction (SC)

Additional qualitative/behavioral observations:
2 circumlocutions and 1 semantic paraphasia

Figure 5.7. Subtest 6: Naming. *Examinee:* 16-year-old 10th-grade male tested 1 month status post ejection from car (no seatbelt)—right subarachnoid and subdural hemorrhages.

- Credit correct responses according to scoring criteria as presented in the right-hand column of the Test Form. These point values were determined by IRT procedures.
- Add earned scores for Total Naming Ability Score.
- Record time to administer.

See Figure 5.7 for an example of scoring of the Naming subtest.

Subtest 7: Story Retelling—Immediate

This test requires examinees to listen to a grade-appropriate story that is read aloud by examiners and then to immediately repeat the story exactly as it was read to them.

Special Instructions

- This subtask requires a verbal response; therefore, it cannot be administered to individuals who cannot speak.
- Three stories are provided: one for Grades 1–3, one for Grades 4–7, one for Grades 8–11.
- Only the story appropriate for the examinee's grade level is read.

Recording and Scoring Subtest Responses

- Story elements and any acceptable variations of each story are listed in the Test Form.
- Check off story elements as they are recalled/spoken by examinees.
- Space is provided for recording variations from the target stories.
- Identify each correct story element:

  Count acceptable semantic substitutions as correct (e.g., "rubbish" or "garbage" for *trash*).

  Do not count variations that change the meaning (e.g., "street" for *sidewalk*).

  Count pronouns as correct, but at first mention, the examinee must use the characters' proper names (e.g., *Bobby, Tommy, Daryl, Rochelle*). For example, use of "she" after mentioning "Tommy's mother" is acceptable. If the examinee uses pronouns throughout (never naming the characters), only the first pronoun (rather than the character's name) does not receive credit.

  Count items told out of sequence as correct. Credit correct responses according to scoring criteria as presented in the right-hand column. These point values were determined by IRT procedures.
- Add earned scores for Total Story Retelling—Immediate Ability Score.
- Record time to administer.

See Figure 5.8 for an example of scoring of the Story Retelling—Immediate subtest.

Subtest 8: Yes/No/Maybe

This subtest requires examinees to follow along while examiners read the short stories printed on pages 12–17 in the Stimulus Book and then answer questions about the story. The correct answers for the questions are "yes," "no," or "maybe," depending on the information provided in the stories.

Special Instructions

- This subtest has a practice item for establishing the idea of responding "yes," "no," or "maybe."
- If examinees remain confused even with this prompting, proceed with the subtest and see if the child is able to respond.
- Once examinees demonstrate the ability to respond "yes," "no," or "maybe" on the practice item, proceed with the test stimuli.
- Discontinue if all the items for two consecutive stories are answered incorrectly.
- If examinees cannot respond verbally, print the words *yes*, *no*, and *maybe* on a piece of paper so they can point to the target answer words.

STORY 3 (GRADES 8–11)

Item	**Story Elements** (optional wording)	Ability Score	Item	**Story Elements** (optional wording)	Ability Score
1	Last spring	(4.5)	23	months	~~2.5~~
2	Daryl got (must use proper name to count)	(2.0)	24	Rochelle (she) said	~~4.0~~
3	two	~~3.0~~	25	to her mother	~~4.0~~
4	free	~~4.0~~	26	if you let me go (allow me to go)	~~3.5~~
5	tickets to	(1.5)	27	and pick us up afterwards	~~1.0~~
6	outdoor	~~5.0~~	28	I promise	~~2.5~~
7	rock	(2.5)	29	to babysit	~~2.5~~
8	concert	(0.5)	30	my sister	~~5.0~~
9	so he asked	(2.5)	31	six times	~~5.0~~
10	his friend	(3.0)	32	both parents	~~5.0~~
11	Rochelle (must use proper name to count)	(3.0)	33	agreed	~~5.0~~
12	to go	(3.5)	34	ten	~~4.0~~
13	with him	(4.0)	35	minutes	~~3.5~~
14	Daryl (he) said	~~3.0~~	36	after the kids	~~1.0~~
15	to his father	~~2.0~~	37	were dropped off	~~2.5~~
16	if you let me go	~~3.0~~	38	it began to "pour" (rain)	(2.0)
17	to the concert	~~3.5~~	39	the concert	~~3.0~~
18	with Rochelle (her)	(3.5)	40	was cancelled	~~5.5~~
19	and drive us (there) (give us a ride)	~~4.0~~	41	the kids (they)	~~2.0~~
20	I will take out	~~2.0~~	42	couldn't believe it (**not**—they were mad)	~~5.5~~
21	the trash (garbage)	~~3.0~~	43	would still have to	~~2.0~~
22	three	~~2.5~~	44	keep their promises (do their jobs)	~~2.0~~

Time to administer: 4.5 min. **Subtotal Score 1** 30.5 / 65.5

Subtotal Score 2 2.0 / 73.0
Subtotal Score 1 30.5 / 65.5
TOTAL STORY RETELLING—IMMEDIATE ABILTY SCORE 32.5 / 138.5

Behavioral observations: (Abbreviations may be used next to items where they apply.)

___ Repetition of instructions (Rep)	___ Perseveration (P)	___ No response (NR)
___ Attention reminder required (Attn)	___ Delayed response (5+ sec) (DR)	___ I don't know (IDK)
___ Prompt to reestablish set (Prompt)	___ Unintelligible response (UnR)	___ Self-correction (SC)

Additional qualitative/behavioral observations:

Primacy effect with most points earned for elements occurring early in story, none in middle, and only one at story conclusion. Reflected in score—30.5 of 32.5 points earned for first half of story.

Figure 5.8. Subtest 7: Story Retelling—Immediate. *Examinee*: 15-year, 10-month-old male in Grade 9 tested 1 month post onset of traumatic brain injury from a head slam on floor during a school fight—punctate left frontal lobe hemorrhage, small left frontal subdural.

Recording and Scoring Subtest Responses

- Circle the examinee's response to each question as printed in the Test Form.
- Correct answers to questions are printed in boldface.
- Score values as determined by IRT procedures appear in the right-hand column of the Test Form.
- Add earned scores for Total Yes/No/Maybe Ability Score.
- Record time to administer.

See Figure 5.9 for an example of scoring of the Yes/No/Maybe subtest.

Short Story 1 (Turn to page 14 in the Stimulus Book. *Note:* This story has only three questions.)			
The kids ran after the blue ice cream truck. It turned the corner before they could catch it.			
Item	**Questions**	**Responses**	**Ability Score**
a	*Did the kids chase the ice cream truck?*	(Y) N M	0.5
b	*Did the kids catch the truck before it turned the corner?*	Y (N) M	0.5
c	*Was the ice cream truck red?*	Y (N) M	0.5
		Story 1 Ability Score	1.5 / 1.5

Short Story 2 (Turn to page 15 in the Stimulus Book.)			
"What I did on my summer vacation" is the topic the teacher makes her class write about on the first day of school every year. When school started a month ago, the teacher gave her usual first writing assignment.			
Item	**Questions**	**Responses**	**Ability Score**
a	*Did the teacher ask her class to write about their summer vacations?*	(Y) N M	0.5
b	*Was the Middle East the first writing topic of the year?*	Y (N) M	~~3.5~~
c	*Did school start last week?*	Y (N) M	~~1.0~~
d	*Did all of the students take a trip on their summer vacations?*	Y N (M)	~~2.0~~
		Story 2 Ability Score	0.5 / 7.0

Short Story 3 (Turn to page 16 in the Stimulus Book.)			
Immanuel was the first one of a small group of boys in his class who could dunk a basketball.			
Item	**Questions**	**Responses**	**Ability Score**
a	*Could Immanuel jump the highest in class?*	Y N (M)	1.0
b	*Could some of the other boys dunk a basketball?*	(Y) N M	~~2.5~~
c	*Could all of the boys in Immanuel's class dunk a basketball?*	Y (N) M	~~2.5~~
d	*Was Immanuel the best basketball player in his class?*	Y N (M)	~~2.0~~
		Story 3 Ability Score	1.0 / 8.0

Short Story 4 (Turn to page 17 in the Stimulus Book.)			
Mary and Todd decided they would go to the beach on Saturday even if it was a cloudy day. When they woke up on Saturday, it was sunny.			
Item	**Questions**	**Responses**	**Ability Score**
a	*Did Mary and Todd plan to go to the beach on Saturday if it was cloudy?*	(Y) N M	2.0
b	*Did it rain later on Saturday?*	Y N (M)	4.0
c	*Was it cloudy when Mary and Todd woke up on Saturday?*	Y (N) M	2.5
d	*Was Mary the mother of Todd?*	Y N (M)	~~2.0~~
		Story 4 Ability Score	8.5 / 10.5

Short Story 5 (Turn to page 18 in the Stimulus Book.)			
The scientists observed the insects closely over a 24-hour period, hoping to study their swarming behavior. At that point, the scientists concluded that the insects had been prevented from swarming because of the unusual atmospheric conditions.			
Item	**Questions**	**Responses**	**Ability Score**
a	*Did the insects swarm?*	Y (N) M	~~4.5~~
b	*Did the scientists watch the insects for a full day?*	(Y) N M	0.5
c	*Can atmospheric conditions influence the swarming of insects?*	(Y) N M	2.5
d	*Did the scientists accomplish their original goal?*	Y (N) M	~~4.5~~
Time to Administer 6 min.		**Story 5 Ability Score**	3.0 / 12.0
		TOTAL YES/NO/MAYBE ABILITY SCORE	14.5 / 39.0

Behavioral observations: (Abbreviations may be used next to items where they apply.)

___ Repetition of instructions (Rep)	___ Perseveration (P)	___ No response (NR)
___ Attention reminder required (Attn)	___ Delayed response (5+ sec) (DR)	___ I don't know (IDK)
___ Prompt to reestablish set (Prompt)	___ Unintelligible response (UnR)	___ Self-correction (SC)

Additional qualitative/behavioral observations:

Tendency to say "maybe" when unsure of answers.

Figure 5.9. Subtest 8: Yes/No/Maybe. *Examinee:* 6-year, 6-month-old male in first grade tested 3 days post being slammed from behind by another child—right temporal depressed skull fracture.

Subtest 9: Picture Recall

This subtest has two components: 1) recalling and drawing from memory the picture of the skateboarder used for Subtest 6 (Naming) and 2) signing or "autographing" the picture.

Special Instructions

- Use the page of the Test Form designated for drawing and autographing the picture.
- Be ready with a black pen (preferably felt-tipped with a fine point) for examinees to draw and write. Never use a pencil with an eraser.
- Let examinees continue drawing/writing as long as they are actively drawing/writing.

Recording and Scoring Subtest Responses

Qualitative examination of pictures may offer insight as to other brain processes and strategies employed in addition to ability to incidentally remember a picture and its details.

- Count all picture elements (listed on the Test Form) that are recognizable in context.
- If an element is not recognizable, ask the examinee "What is this?" and give credit if it is a correct element.
- If the examinee is unable to hold a pen to draw a recognizable picture, ask for a description, write down what the child says, and score recalled elements.
- If the child cannot move to write his or her name, ask for a spelling. All letters in the name must be correct (in context) to earn a score.
- Credit correct responses according to scoring criteria as presented in the right-hand column. These points were determined by IRT procedures. Add all earned points to compute Total Picture Recall Ability Score.
- Record time to administer.

See Figure 5.10 for an example of scoring of the Picture Recall subtest.

Subtest 10: Story Retelling—Delayed

This subtest requires examinees to recall and retell the grade–appropriate story that was read to them in Subtest 7.

Special Instructions

- See the special instructions for Subtest 7: Story Retelling—Immediate.

Item	Picture Recall	Ability Score
1	Picture of a boy	~~1.5~~
2	Skateboard	(3.0)
3	Hat / Baseball cap	~~5.5~~
4	Boots / Shoes	~~5.5~~
5	Star	(6.0)
6	Chain / ID tags / Dog tags / Necklace	(6.0)
7	Band-Aid	~~7.0~~
8	Shorts	~~7.5~~
	Picture Recall Subtotal	15.0 / 42.0

Item	Signature	Ability Score
1	First name	(0.5)
2	Last name	(3.0)

Signature Subtotal 3.5 / 3.5

Picture Recall Subtotal 15.0 / 42.0

TOTAL PICTURE RECALL ABILITY SCORE 18.5 / 45.5

Time to administer: 4 min.

Hand used: ___ L ✓ R

Behavioral observations: (Abbreviations may be used next to items where they apply.)

___ Repetition of instructions (Rep)	___ Perseveration (P)	___ No response (NR)
___ Attention reminder required (Attn)	___ Delayed response (5+ sec) (DR)	___ I don't know (IDK)
___ Prompt to reestablish set (Prompt)	___ Unintelligible response (UnR)	___ Self-correction (SC)

Additional qualitative/behavioral observations:

Curious omission of lower body although recalls two details (chain, star) on upper body and skateboard as unconnected element.

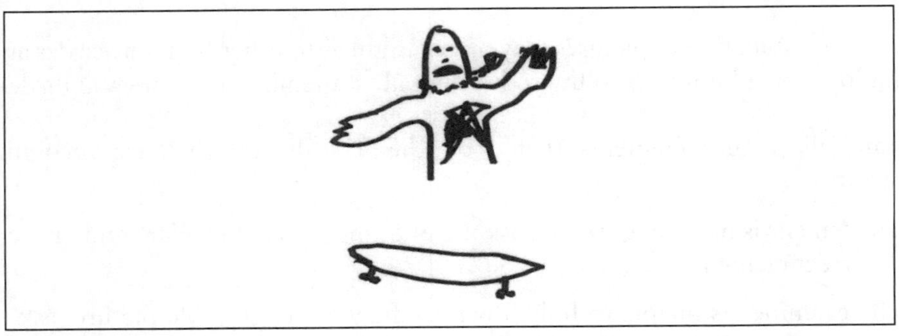

Figure 5.10. Subtest 9: Picture Recall. *Examinee:* 8-year, 2-month-old male in third grade tested 6 weeks post being struck on the head by a blunt instrument. Computed tomography (CT) showed cerebral edema. (*Note:* Same boy as Figure 5.5. Signature removed for confidentiality.)

Recording and Scoring Subtest Responses

- As the child retells the story, check items recalled correctly or record verbatim any content variations in the story produced.
- Identify each correct item.
- Count acceptable semantic substitutions as correct (e.g., "rubbish" or "garbage" for *trash).*
- Do not count variations that change the meaning (e.g., "street" for *sidewalk*).
- Count pronouns as correct, but at first mention, the examinee must use the characters' proper names (e.g., *Bobby, Tommy, Daryl, Rochelle*). For example, use of "she" after mentioning "Tommy's mother" is acceptable. If the examinee uses pronouns throughout (never naming the characters), only the first pronoun (rather than the character's name) does not receive credit.
- Count items told out of sequence as correct.

STORY 3 (GRADES 8–11)

Item	**Story Elements** (optional wording)	Ability Score	Item	**Story Elements** (optional wording)	Ability Score
1	Last spring	~~4.0~~	23	months	~~2.5~~
2	Daryl got (must use proper name to count) *boy*	~~2.0~~	24	Rochelle (she) said *Rosie*	~~2.5~~
3	two	~~2.5~~	25	to her mother	(1.5)
4	free	~~4.0~~	26	if you let me go (allow me to go)	(3.0)
5	tickets to	(1.0)	27	and pick us up afterwards	~~3.0~~
6	outdoor	~~4.5~~	28	I promise	~~2.5~~
7	rock	(1.5)	29	to babysit	~~1.0~~
8	concert	(0.5)	30	my sister	~~2.5~~
9	so he asked	~~2.0~~	31	six times	~~2.5~~
10	his friend	~~2.5~~	32	both parents	~~4.0~~
11	Rochelle (must use proper name to count)	~~2.5~~	33	agreed	~~3.5~~
12	to go	~~2.5~~	34	ten	~~3.5~~
13	with him	~~0.5~~	35	minutes	~~3.5~~
14	Daryl (he) said *boy*	~~2.5~~	36	after the kids	~~3.0~~
15	to his father *parent*	~~1.5~~	37	were dropped off	~~3.0~~
16	if you let me go	~~3.0~~	38	it began to "pour" (rain)	(1.0)
17	to the concert	~~4.0~~	39	the concert	~~1.0~~
18	with Rochelle (her) *Rosie*	~~4.5~~	40	was cancelled	~~1.5~~
19	and drive us (there) (give us a ride)	~~3.0~~	41	the kids (they)	~~3.0~~
20	I will take out	~~1.5~~	42	couldn't believe it (**not**—they were mad)	~~0.5~~
21	the trash (garbage)	~~1.0~~	43	would still have to	~~1.5~~
22	three	~~2.5~~	44	keep their promises (do their jobs)	~~1.5~~

Time to administer: *3 min*. **Subtotal Score 1** *3.0* / 56.5

Subtotal Score 2 *5.5* / 54.5
Subtotal Score 1 *3.0* / 56.5
TOTAL STORY RETELLING—DELAYED ABILTY SCORE *8.5* / 111.0

Behavioral observations: (Abbreviations may be used next to items where they apply.)

___ Repetition of instructions (Rep)	___ Perseveration (P)	___ No response (NR)
___ Attention reminder required (Attn)	___ Delayed response (5+ sec) (DR)	___ I don't know (IDK)
___ Prompt to reestablish set (Prompt)	___ Unintelligible response (UnR)	___ Self-correction (SC)

Additional qualitative/behavioral observations:

Compared to Story Retelling—Immediate—scores 8.5 vs. 32.5—loss of information but now recalls two items from mid-story.

Figure 5.11. Subtest 10: Story Retelling. *Examinee*: 15-year, 10-month-old male in Grade 9 tested 1 month post onset of traumatic brain injury from a head slam on floor during a school fight—punctate left frontal lobe hemorrhage, small left frontal subdural. (*Note:* Same boy as Figure 5.8.)

- Add points for correct items to compute Total Story Retelling—Delayed Ability Score. These points were determined by IRT procedures.
- Record time to administer.

See Figure 5.11 for an example of scoring of the Story Retelling—Delayed subtest.

CONCLUSION

This chapter provided instructions for administering and scoring the PTBI. Chapter 6 contains validity and reliability information as well as information concerning analysis of test bias.

6

Evidence-Based Practice (Technical Analyses)

Examiners need to know that the interpretations they make are supported by data-based evidence. In this chapter, we review the types of questions examiners should ask about the nature of any test, which will inform their conclusions about test performance. Therefore, this section covers validity and reliability information as well as information concerning analysis of test bias.

We continue to use the concept of constrained and unconstrained skills (cf. Paris, 2005) to interpret results. To review, *constrained* subtests tap skills that develop relatively early in development (e.g., knowing one's name, naming common items). *Unconstrained* subtests tap skills that tend to show continued refinement over a wide range of ages. The PTBI contains both types of subtests, and the statistical results are presented separately for each type. A question and answer framework is used to describe the evidence base related to various clinical questions about the nature of the PTBI.

EVIDENCE FOR CONSTRUCT-IDENTIFICATION VALIDITY

Question 1: How do I interpret the criterion categories?

The categories of performance for each age are based on the performance of the group of children without brain injuries selected to represent the general population. The percentages of these children whose scores fell into each of the four criterion categories is provided in Table 6.1. As this table shows, most scores fell into the High performance category. The differences in the percentages of children classified into the different performance categories reflects naturally occurring differences in the range of performance that children in the general population show in these different skill areas.

Technical Notes

Scores from 103 children (57 girls, 46 boys) were classified against the criterion categories for this source of evidence. They ranged in age from 6 to 16 years, with an average age

Table 6.1. Classification of scores of children without brain injuries into performance categories

	Performance categories			
Subscale	Very Low	Low	Moderate	High
1. Orientation	0%	6%	19%	75%
2. Following Commands	7%	8%	2%	83%
3. Word Fluency	3%	20%	25%	53%
4. What Goes Together	2%	1%	19%	78%
5. Digit Span	2%	6%	30%	62%
6. Naming	0%	4%	3%	93%
7. Story Retelling—Immediate	2%	10%	28%	60%
8. Yes/No/Maybe	0%	5%	18%	77%
9. Picture Recall	0%	5%	35%	60%
10. Story Retelling—Delayed	0%	3%	20%	77%

of 9 years, 11 months. No child had been diagnosed with a brain injury (TBI or ABI). Note that children were not screened for other conditions that occur in the general population that could affect performance (e.g., learning disability). Therefore, this group is intended to reflect the non–brain-injured general population. Sixty-nine of the children were white, twenty-three were African American, four were Hispanic, two were reported as "other," and one was Asian. Race was not reported for four children. Of the children, 86 were right-handed, 9 were left-handed, and handedness was not reported for 8 children.

Question 2: How do I know the PTBI is testing skills that are relevant to the types of deficits shown by children with neurological disorders?

As Table 6.2 shows, the typically developing children received higher ability scores on all subtests compared with the ABI group. Children with TBI scored significantly lower than their peers without brain injuries on all seven subtests that assess unconstrained skills and two of the constrained skills subtests. The ability scores on the constrained skills subtests were close to ceiling for all three groups; therefore, these subtests are most useful clinically for children with severe impairments. It is also the case that the children with ABI differed from their peers with TBI on four of the subtests, indicating that the pattern of deficits is not necessarily the same for both groups. These data support *construct-identification validity* (Anastasi & Urbina, 1997).

Technical Notes

Ninety-nine children's scores were compared for this source of evidence. Thirty-three children were included in each of the three groups (TBI, ABI, typical). These children were matched by age (mean age of 10 years, 7 months; range 6–16 years) and gender (14 males, 19 females per group). A variety of racial/ethnic groups were included (TBI: 26 white, 7 minority; ABI: 17 white, 16 minority; Typical: 22 white, 11 minority). The majority of the children in each group were right-handed (TBI: 27 right-handed; ABI: 27 right-handed, typical: 25 right-handed). Ability scores were tested using t tests with statistical significance at $p < .05$.

Table 6.2. Raw score means (standard deviations) for matched groups of children with traumatic brain injury (TBI; $n = 33$), other acquired brain injury (ABI; $n = 33$), and typically developing children (Typical, $n = 33$).

	Constrained skills			Unconstrained skills						
Category	1. Orientation	2. Following Commands	6. Naming	3. Word Fluency	4. What Goes Together	5. Digit Span	7. Story Retelling —Immediate	8. Yes/No/ Maybe	9. Picture Recall	10. Story Retelling —Delayed
TBI	30.8[a, b]	14.7	12.18[a,b]	20.37[a,b]	49.51[b]	28.50[b]	45.63[b]	20.57[b]	29.39[a,b]	25.97[b]
	(8.25)	(1.14)	(0.79)	(9.11)	(23.59)	(21.7)	(33.65)	(7.26)	(12.66)	(16.28)
ABI	24.94[a,c]	13.65[c]	11.27[a,c]	14.97[a,c]	52.62[c]	22.08[c]	39.67[c]	18.28[c]	18.70[a,c]	26.09[c]
	(6.75)	(2.45)	(2.35)	(9.60)	(25.32)	(20.71)	(36.01)	(8.13)	(14.39)	(22.98)
Typical	36.02[b,c]	14.90[c]	12.40[b,c]	27.27[b,c]	69.02[b,c]	40.75[b,c]	61.33[b,c]	24.03[b,c]	34.42[b,c]	43.90[b,c]
	(5.29)	(0.54)	(0.38)	(7.74)	(19.83)	(20.40)	(34.53)	(7.37)	(8.31)	(19.91)
Total possible	38.0	15.0	12.5	No limit	100.5	82.5	(1) 51.5 (2) 142.5 (3) 138.5	39.0	45.5	(1) 51.5 (2) 83.0 (3) 111.0

[a]Significant difference between typical and TBI and ABI groups ($p < .05$).
[b]Significant difference between TBI and Typical groups ($p < .05$).
[c]Significant difference between ABI and Typical groups ($p < .05$).
Note: There are three possible point values (one for each story) on Subtests 7 and 10 .

Table 6.3. Correlations between the PTBI subtests and two indices of severity of injury

Scale	Unconstrained skills						
	3. Word Fluency	4. What Goes Together	5. Digit Span	7. Story Retelling—Immediate	8. Yes/No/Maybe	9. Picture Recall	10. Story Retelling—Delayed
Glasgow Coma Scale	.30	.58[a]	–.05	.34[a]	.46[a]	.49[a]	.43[a]
Rancho Los Amigos Scale	.44[a]	.56[a]	.03	.37[a]	.40[a]	.50[a]	.41[a]

[a]Statistically significant correlations at $p < .05$.

Question 3: Are scores on the PTBI related to the degree of severity of the brain injury for children with TBI?

To address this issue, we correlated the scores on the unconstrained skills subtests of PTBI with scores on the Glasgow Coma Scale (Teasdale & Jennett, 1974) and the Rancho Los Amigos Scale (Hagen, Malkmus, & Durham, 1979). These two scales are frequently used to index severity of brain injury. We did not correlate the constrained skills subtests because the lack of variability in scores even in children with TBI and ABI (see Table 6.2) made this type of statistical analysis inappropriate. As Table 6.3 shows, the scores on most subtests of the PTBI are correlated with severity. However, the degree of correlation is such that the scores of individual PTBI subtests can diverge from these two scales in noteworthy ways for any given individual. This analysis provides a form of criterion-related validity and supports construct-identification validity.

Technical Notes

Thirty-eight individuals (14 females, 24 males) with TBI received both the Glasgow Coma Scale and the Rancho Los Amigos Scale at or near the time of testing. The mean age of these children was 12 years, 9 months (range 7–16 years). Twenty of the children were white, and eighteen were members of minority groups. Thirty-six individuals were right-handed. Pearson product-moment correlations were calculated between each of the subtests of the PTBI and the two scales that index severity. Note that the correlation between the Glasgow Coma Scale and the Rancho Los Amigo Scale was .46.

Question 4: How do I know that the scores I obtain actually reflect a child's ability on the skills tapped by the subtest?

State-of-the-art methods of estimating a child's ability require computation that is often complex and/or time-consuming. Therefore, it was important to have a scoring method that accurately estimated a child's ability but could be computed with relative ease. It also was important to establish that this simple method of calculating a child's ability is close to the ability level that more sophisticated statistical methods would produce.

The ability scores based on the difficulty of the items the child passed or failed were compared with the modeled estimate of child ability using IRT statistical procedures. As

Table 6.4. Correlations between calculated ability scores and statistically modeled ability levels

Constrained skills			Unconstrained skills						
1. Orientation	2. Following Commands	6. Naming	3. Word Fluency	4. What Goes Together	5. Digit Span	7. Story Retelling —Immediate	8. Yes/No/ Maybe	9. Picture Recall	10. Story Retelling —Delayed
.94	.96	.96	1.00[a]	.75	.93	1) .94 2) .98 3) .90	.97	.94	1) .95 2) .92 3) .85

[a]Because of its open-ended scoring (number of words produced), the Word Fluency subtest was not appropriate for analysis using IRT procedures. For this subtest, raw score = ability score.

Note: There are three possible point values (one for each story) on Subtests 7 and 10.

Table 6.4 illustrates, there was a very high correlation between the calculated ability score and the modeled ability of the children tested.

Technical Notes

The standardization sample of 257 children was used for this analysis. Children were between the ages of 6 and 16. Their demographic characteristics are reported in Tables 3.1 and 3.2. Their ability scores were calculated based on the instructions in the test manual. Pearson product-moment correlations were used to correlate calculated ability scores with the ability estimates obtained through IRT methods for each child. IRT methods used a Rasch model to estimate item difficulty and child ability based on subtest performance.

Question 5: When I am looking at performance across subtests, what should I know about how related the different subtests are?

This question addresses another aspect of construct-identification validity. To answer this question, we can consult two sources of data. The first is simple correlations between subtests, and the second is a more sophisticated correlation-based technique known as *factor analysis*. Remember that for the three constrained skills subtests (Subtest 1: Orientation; Subtest 2: Following Commands; Subtest 6: Naming), performance was at ceiling for most children in all three groups (see Table 6.2). Because of this, we excluded these three subtests from these analyses. The lack of variability in the children's scores makes these subtests inappropriate for correlation-based techniques.

Table 6.5 shows the correlations among subtests. As expected, all subtests correlate to some degree because all subtests require the use of language to some degree (even Subtest 9: Picture Recall). There are also some high correlations that one would expect. For example, scores on Subtest 10: Story Retelling—Delayed are strongly correlated with scores on the initial Subtest 7: Story Retelling—Immediate. However, unless you have specific comparisons in mind, it is difficult to make sense of a correlation matrix. For this reason, we used factor analysis to determine the extent to which the scores on various subtests seem

Table 6.5. Correlations among total ability scores for unconstrained skills subtests

	3. Word Fluency	4. What Goes Together	5. Digit Span	7. Story Retelling—Immediate	8. Yes/No/Maybe	9. Picture Recall	10. Story Retelling—Delayed
3. Word Fluency	1.00	.59	.45	.56	.55	.57	.60
4. What Goes Together	.59	1.00	.36	.56	.54	.56	.54
5. Digit Span	.45	.36	1.00	.29	.30	.37	.25
7. Story Retelling—Immediate	.56	.56	.29	1.00	.63	.49	.79
8. Yes/No/Maybe	.55	.54	.30	.63	1.00	.44	.59
9. Picture Recall	.57	.56	.37	.49	.44	1.00	.48
10. Story Retelling—Delayed	.60	.55	.25	.79	.59	.48	1.00

Note: All correlations are statistically significant.

Table 6.6. Factor loadings for the unconstrained skill subtests of the PTBI

	Factor 1	Factor 2	Factor 3
7. Story Retelling—Immediate	**0.86**	0.27	0.17
10. Story Retelling—Delayed	**0.86**	0.27	0.07
8. Yes/No/Maybe	**0.77**	0.22	0.23
3. Word Fluency	0.47	0.57	0.39
4. What Goes Together	0.45	0.67	0.20
9. Picture Recall	0.23	**0.87**	0.17
5. Digit Span	0.11	0.17	**0.97**

to coalesce, suggesting some common set of skills may be needed for the subtests that belong to a particular factor.

Table 6.6 shows the factor loadings for the seven unconstrained subtests. *Factor loadings* are the degree to which subtest scores correlate with the overarching factor. As this table illustrates, the seven subtests seem to reflect three common factors. The three subtests (Subtests 7, 8, and 10) that require language processing at the sentence/discourse level load on Factor 1. The strongest loading for Factor 2 is for Picture Recall (Subtest 9). What Goes Together (Subtest 4) also loads on this factor. These two subtests require mental organization and integration (semantic and visual). Factor 3 includes only Digit Span (Subtest 5), which requires attention and immediate memory. Word Fluency (Subtest 3) and What Goes Together (Subtest 4) load fairly evenly on all three factors, indicating commonality with skill sets that cross cognitive and linguistic domains.

Technical Notes

Exploratory factor analysis was completed on the ability scores of 257 children between the ages of 6 and 16. Their demographic characteristics are reported in Tables 3.1 and 3.2. We used an initial unrotated principal components analysis and examined the scree plot to determine the likely number of factors. Factors were rotated using a Varimax procedure. We considered both two-factor and three-factor solutions. The three-factor solution provided a more meaningful grouping of subtests and was retained. The difference between the two solutions affected only the Picture Recall subtest, which in the two-factor solution did not clearly load primarily on either of the first two factors.

Question 6: Do scores on subtests designed to assess unconstrained (developmental) skills correlate with age?

We expected subtests that reflected unconstrained skills to show age-related development because, by definition, unconstrained skills develop over a protracted time period. However, the presence of a neurological disorder can disrupt skill acquisition. Therefore, we examined this issue only for typically developing children. As Table 6.2 shows, performance on the constrained skills subtests were near ceiling for most children. This made conducting correlations inappropriate for these subtests because of the highly restricted variability in scores. In contrast, all unconstrained skill subtests showed statistically significant age-related change. This is additional converging evidence for construct-identification validity. Table 6.7 shows age correlations for unconstrained skills.

Table 6.7. Age correlations for unconstrained skills

	3. Word Fluency	4. What Goes Together	5. Digit Span	7. Story Retelling—Immediate	8. Yes/No/Maybe	9. Picture Recall	10. Story Retelling—Delayed
Total possible score	N/A	100.5	82.5	1) 51.5 2) 142.5 3) 138.5	39.0	45.5	1) 51.5 2) 83.0 3) 111.0
Mean score	28.1	66.3	38.7	57.3	37.6	33.4	42.2
Age correlation	.51[a]	.39[a]	.47[a]	.70[a]	.68[a]	.54[a]	.66[a]

[a]Statistically significant at $p < .05$.

Note: There are three possible point values (one for each story) on Subtests 7 and 10.

Technical notes

Seventy-seven (29 male, 48 female) typically developing children between the ages of 6 and 16 years (mean 9 years, 9 months) were studied. Sixty-two were white, and fifteen were members of various minority groups. Their demographic information can be found in Table 3.2. Sixty-seven of the children were right handed, seven were left-handed, one was ambidexterous, and handedness was not reported for two children. Pearson product-moment correlations were calculated for age and each of the PTBI subtests, and statistical significance was set at $p < .05$.

EVIDENCE FOR RELIABILITY

Reliability data indicate how likely the test is to yield stable information about the child. There are several forms of reliability, and each can be used to address different concerns that a clinician may have when interpreting a test score. These are explained next.

Question 7: How do I know whether change is due to real improvement or just fluctuation that would occur from one test session to the next?

To answer this question, one would have to know that children who are neurologically stable (i.e., typically developing children) receive highly similar scores when tested more than once. This is known as *test–retest reliability*. Test–retest reliability values range from 0 (no correspondence between scores obtained at two different test session) to 1.00 (identical scores obtained by all children at two different test sessions). Note that the test–retest reliability coefficient was the basis for calculating the standard error of measurement (*SEM*). Therefore, the *SEM*, which is used to track change, accounts for normal test-to-test fluctuation. Table 6.8 shows test–retest reliability for each of the 10 subtests.

Technical Notes

Test–retest reliability was evaluated on 40 children between the ages of 6 and 16 years (mean 10 years). No child had a diagnosis of TBI or ABI. Twenty-three of the children were

African American, twelve were white, three were Hispanic, and two were described as "other." All children were retested after 3–6 weeks (average 32 days, range of 23 to 45 days). Test–retest reliability was determined using a Pearson product-moment correlation calculated on the ability scores for each of the subtests. Correlations were adjusted for restricted range using the method of Gulliksen (1950). All correlations are statistically significant at $p < .05$.

Question 8: How do I know that test scores are not influenced by differences in opinion about how to score the test items?

To answer this question, we would need to have two people independently score tests given to a group of children. This is known as *interrater reliability.* Interrater reliability can be calculated by computing the percent agreement in scoring by two examiners on an item-by-item basis. This is called *point-to-point agreement.* Alternatively, it can be calculated based on the total ability score for each subtest. The latter is based on the correlation between two sets of ability scores obtained from two examiners. In this case, interrater reliability values can vary between 0 (no correspondence between scores obtained by different raters) and 1 (perfect agreement among scores by different raters). Table 6.9 shows interrater reliability for the PTBI subtests.

Technical Notes

Interrater reliability was evaluated on 41 children (19 male, 22 female) who were between the ages of 6 and 17 years (mean 11 years, 8 months). The racial and ethnic characteristics of the children included 15 white children, 17 African American children, 3 Hispanic children, and 6 described as "other." These children included 15 with a diagnosis of TBI, 15 with a diagnosis of ABI, and 11 without brain injury. Tests were originally scored by 14 clinicians. Tests were rescored by a research assistant using the responses recorded verbatim at the time of testing. All raters scored the test items based on the written instructions available on the test protocols. Point-to-point values were calculated based on the percentage of items scored identically by the pair of raters. Correlations were calculated using Pearson product-moment correlation applied to the raw scores for the subtest and total test scores. All correlations are statistically significant at $p < .05$.

EVIDENCE FOR MINIMIZATION OF BIAS

Bias is identified when one group performs differently than another. Therefore, evidence of bias can be assessed empirically. Bias is a concern when interpretation of test performance is influenced by factors irrelevant to the purpose of the test. Next is a discussion of several areas where bias might be a concern and how potential bias was evaluated.

Question 9: What is the evidence that bias has been minimized?

We examined multiple sources of bias to be sure that potential irrelevant influences were either absent or were controlled in ways that would not affect the types of interpretation that examiners would wish to make about test performance.

Table 6.8. Test–retest reliability

	Constrained skills						Unconstrained skills													
	1. Orientation		2. Following Commands		6. Naming		3. Word Fluency		4. What Goes Together		5. Digit Span		7. Story Retelling —Immediate		8. Yes/No/ Maybe		9. Picture Recall		10. Story Retelling —Delayed	
	Time 1	Time 2	Time 1	Time 2	Time 1	Time 2	Time 1	Time 2	Time 1	Time 2	Time 1	Time 2	Time 1	Time 2	Time 1	Time 2	Time 1	Time 2	Time 1	Time 2
Mean	35.6	36.6	12.0	12.0	12.5	12.5	27.2	29.6	70.4	80.2	33.4	31.7	58.8	56.3	25.2	26.1	31.9	35.6	37.3	39.9
SD	4.4	3.1	3.38	3.45	0	0	7.9	7.5	21.7	19.5	14.0	13.6	38.1	31.8	8.0	7.5	9.5	10.6	17.9	20.2
Adjusted *r*	.88		.99		1.00[a]		.80		.81		.84		1) .83 2) .79 3) .84		.80		.75		1) .80 2) .88 3) .77	

Key: SD, standard deviation.

[a]All subjects scored at the ceiling of 12.5 at both test sessions. Therefore, there was perfect agreement and an *r* cannot be estimated.

Note: There are three possible point values (one for each story) on Subtests 7 and 10.

Table 6.9. Interrater reliability

	Constrained skills			Unconstrained skills						
	1. Orientation	2. Following Commands	6. Naming	3. Word Fluency	4. What Goes Together	5. Digit Span	7. Story Retelling —Immediate	8. Yes/No/ Maybe	9. Picture Recall	10 Story Retelling —Delayed
Point-to-point agreement	99%	99%	100%	100%	98%	100%	100%	100%	99%	100%
Correlation	.98	1.00	1.00	1.00	.99	.99	1.00	1.00	.99	1.00

Diagnostic Category

The most critical aspect concerning bias is whether one group of children would be classified differently than another based on aspects of their background (e.g., gender, minority status) other than brain injury. To examine this issue, we considered the rate at which typically developing children were classified into the different criterion categories (i.e., Very Low to High performance). Table 6.10 illustrates that white and minority children's scores fell into similar classification strata, with the greatest number of both white and minority children falling into the High performance category.

Technical Notes

Data from 70 white and 31 minority children were analyzed for Table 6.10. Minority children included 24 African American children, 4 Hispanic children, 1 Asian child, and 2 children described as "other." Children ranged in age from 6 to 16 years (mean 9 years). Scores were classified using the age-appropriate tables in Appendix A.

Analysis of Item Bias in Subtests Tapping Unconstrained Skills

Many test manuals suggest that a diverse composition of the normative group is evidence against test bias. We have included such diversity in our criterion-referenced sample (see Table 3.2); however, bias can occur even when racial, ethnic, and gender diversity is represented in the test sample. Therefore, it is important to explicitly evaluate test items for bias statistically. Item bias can be identified when children of similar abilities nonetheless do not perform on individual items in a similar manner. We evaluated the test items for this possibility using a technique called *differential item functioning (DIF)* at each phase of the development of the PTBI. Candidate items that showed evidence of DIF for males versus females, whites versus racial/ethnic minorities, and monolingual versus bilingual speakers were excluded from the final test.

Table 6.11 reports correlation coefficients for item difficulty levels established for different subgroups of children. As the differences in item difficulty for each subgroup suggest, performance was relatively similar for each subgroup for which bias was assessed. Furthermore, correlations closer to 1.00 reflected smaller differences between the subgroups in terms of how easy or difficult the children found the items. The lowest correlations occurred for minority or bilingual children on the two subtests that involved story retelling (Subtests 7 and 10). This is not unexpected in that narrative structures are culturally dependent (Westby, 1994). Therefore, we examined performance by broad racial/ethnic subgroups when setting the criterion scores to assure that children in "minority" subgroups were not disadvantaged.

Technical Notes

For the DIF analyses, we used the 257 children described in Tables 3.1 and 3.2. We employed a delta plot approach (Angoff & Ford, 1973) in evaluating DIF between the subgroups of children. DIF can produce chance differences on individual items; therefore, we also looked at the overall performance on the subtest.

Table 6.10. Classification of white and minority children in terms of performance criterion categories

	White (n = 70)				Minority (n = 31)			
Subscale	Very Low	Low	Moderate	High	Very Low	Low	Moderate	High
1. Orientation	1	4	11	54	0	5	6	20
2. Following Commands	3	4	1	62	5	2	1	23
3. Word Fluency	3	12	15	40	0	6	12	13
4. What Goes Together	1	0	12	57	1	2	6	22
5. Digit Span	2	4	17	47	0	5	11	15
6. Naming	0	4	2	64	0	0	1	30
7. Story Retelling—Immediate[a]	2	4	13	49	0	6	11	13
8. Yes/No/Maybe[a]	0	4	14	52	0	2	6	21
9. Picture Recall	0	1	20	49	0	0	14	17
10. Story Retelling—Delayed	0	3	11	56	0	0	9	22

[a]Scores unavailable for some children.

Table 6.11. Item difficulty differences and correlations for subgroups of children on the PTBI

Item	Boys vs. Girls		White vs. Minority		English monlingual vs. bilingual	
	Mean (*SD*) difference	Correlation	Mean (*SD*) difference	Correlation	Mean (*SD*) difference	Correlation
4. What Goes Together	.03 (.47)	.91	.00 (.52)	.96	.03 (.47)	.95
5. Digit Span	.03 (.87)	.99	.05 (.47)	1.00	.02 (1.15)	.98
7. Story Retelling—Immediate	.01 (.64)	.87	.08 (.83)	.81	.10 (1.16)	.79
8. Yes/No/Maybe	.04 (.40)	.95	.00 (.51)	.89	.02 (.59)	.84
9. Story Retelling—Delayed	.02 (.79)	.82	.10 (.89)	.75	.06 (.95)	.72
10. Picture Recall	.22 (.91)	.96	.08 (.51)	.98	.22 (.78)	.96

Note: Mean difference is the average difference in IRT ability score on subtest items for each group.
Key: SD, standard deviation.

The constrained skills subtests (Subtest 1: Orientation; Subtest 2: Following Commands; Subtest 6: Naming) were not analyzed with DIF. This is because children in all subgroups performed at or near ceiling on these subtests unless they had severe disabilities. This created conditions that were inappropriate for conducting correlational analyses (i.e., restricted ranges, discontinuous distributions). However, because all children were performing at ceiling, it was obvious that there were no meaningful differences by subgroup. An alternate examination of the constrained skills subtests is provided in the next section.

The DIF procedure also was not performed on the Word Fluency subtest. The open-ended nature of scoring for the Word Fluency subtest precluded analysis with DIF procedures.

Analysis of Item Bias in Subtests Tapping Constrained Skills and the Word Fluency Subtest

Table 6.12 shows the subgroup means and standard deviations for those subtests that were inappropriate for DIF analysis. Caution should be applied in interpreting group differences on these subtests because we were unable to equate subgroups for their overall severity, which is a significant advantage for the DIF approach. This being said, the distributions of scores showed a large degree of overlap between subgroups. The largest differences were noted on Word Fluency for minority and bilingual children. This is not surprising because the bilingual children were often also the minority children. In addition, bilingual children

Table 6.12. Means and standard deviations for constrained skills subtests and Word Fluency subtest for subgroups of children

	Boys	Girls	White	Minority	Monolingual English	Bilingual
1. Orientation	26.43	27.13	26.99	25.92	26.98	24.99
	(5.58)	(4.12)	(4.16)	(6.28)	(5.34)	(7.39)
2. Following Commands	14.51	14.81	14.70	14.61	14.64	13.82
	(1.50)	(0.74)	(1.09)	(1.07)	(1.00)	(2.05)
3. Word Fluency	21.30	22.77	21.88	18.38	21.82	16.46
	(9.60)	(11.42)	(9.68)	(9.35)	(11.55)	(8.64)
6. Naming	11.81	12.23	12.88	11.41	11.70	10.71
	(1.59)	(1.39)	(0.97)	(2.84)	(2.50)	(3.35)

may have both a smaller corpus of English vocabulary and more difficulty retrieving English words (e.g., Bedore, Peña, García, & Cortez, 2005; Gollan & Kroll, 2001; Michael & Gollan, 2005; Portocarrero, Burright, & Donovick, 2007). We took this into consideration when setting criterion scores in order to eliminate potential bias from this source.

Technical Notes

The gender comparison used 86 children with TBI, 32 children with ABI, and 52 typically developing children. Girls and boys in each group were matched for age. The race/ethnicity comparison included 76 children with TBI, 20 children with ABI, and 24 typically developing children. Half of the children were white and half belonged to other racial or ethnic minority groups. These included 35 African American children, 2 Asian children, 18 Hispanic children, 1 Native American child, and 4 children identified as "other." Children in the white and minority groups were matched for age. The English monolingual versus bilingual comparison involved 36 children with TBI, 16 with ABI, and 4 typically developing children. Twenty-eight of these children were monolingual English speakers, eighteen were speakers of English and Spanish, and ten spoke English and a language other than Spanish. Children in the English monolingual and bilingual groups were matched for age.

CONCLUSION

This chapter guided examiners through the questions to ask to determine test performance. The evidence base for the PTBI was presented. Chapter 7 provides a case study demonstrating a test and retest of the PTBI.

7

Case Example

In this chapter we present a case example demonstrating a test and retest of the PTBI, including two completed Test Forms. The 14-year-old male, J.D. (a pseudonym), was in 10th grade at the time of the accident. He was tested the first time 28 days post onset of TBI caused by a crash on a mini motor bike. (J.D. was not wearing a helmet.) His Rancho Los Amigos Scale (RLAS) at the time of testing was a VI (confused-appropriate).

J.D. sustained a small left subdural hemorrhage, left frontal and temporal contusions with mass effect, and cerebral edema. He underwent a frontal-parietal craniotomy for decompression. After a short stay in the pediatric intensive care unit (ICU), he was transferred to an acute adolescent unit bed until he was medically and surgically stable. He was then transferred to the pediatric rehabilitation unit, where he remained for 10 weeks, receiving a comprehensive neurorehabilitation program. The second PTBI was administered 5 months post onset when J.D. was being seen for outpatient speech-language therapy.

A general recommendation is for the first administration of the PTBI to be given to the child as a baseline test when he or she is able to follow simple commands and pay attention for a short period of time. Typically, this may be in an ICU or acute care setting. Depending on the child's length of stay in an acute care setting, the PTBI can be administered on a weekly basis in order to monitor recovery. It is also recommended that, if the child is transferred to an inpatient rehabilitation program, the PTBI be administered on admission and then again on discharge in order to monitor recovery and any changes in neurocognitive skills. The PTBI can also be administered in an outpatient clinic setting and used as part of testing for school reentry evaluations along with a neuropsychological test battery. In this case example, J.D. was tested twice with the PTBI: once while he was an inpatient and once in the initial visit of his outpatient therapy program.

REPORTING RESULTS

Clinicians must provide different types of reports depending on the requirements of the institutional setting (e.g., hospital, rehabilitation center, outpatient clinic, school), third party payers (e.g., insurance companies, Medicaid), and purposes of the report (e.g., transition back to school or eligibility for services in school). For demonstration purposes, we have written two kinds of reports regarding J.D.'s test results. The brief summary is the kind of report that would be appropriate for the child's medical record. The longer, more complete summary might be used as a discharge summary for a child returning to school and requiring further testing, including dynamic assessment of recovering abilities.

BRIEF SUMMARY

The Pediatric Test of Brain Injury is a test that assesses neurocognitive and language abilities of children recovering from brain injury. The test is criterion referenced and provides cut-off scores for each subtest that can be used to provide age-related ability ratings, performance classification, and confidence interval ranges (reported on the test protocol in the patient's file). The results of the PTBI administered to J.D. on June 3, 2009, yielded the following ability scores and corresponding performance levels:

1. *Orientation*: 7.5—Very Low performance level.
2. *Following Commands*: 5.0—Very Low
3. *Word Fluency*: 2.0—Very Low
4. *What Goes Together* (vocabulary relationships): 22.5—Very Low
5. *Digit Span*: 82.5—High
6. *Naming*: 4.0—Very Low
7. *Story Retelling—Immediate*: 0—Very Low
8. *Yes/No/Maybe* (language comprehension): 1.0—Very Low
9. *Picture Recall*: 5.0—Very Low
10. *Story Retelling—Delayed*: 0—Very Low
11. *Overall performance rating*: Very Low (except for Digit Span).

In summary, when he was initially tested on June 3, 2009 (1 month post onset), J.D. demonstrated significant deficits in all areas of neurocognition and language, with the exception of short-term numerical recall. J.D.'s overall PTBI performance was within the very low range. The only subtest where he demonstrated high performance was Digit Span. Recommendations at this time include activities to improve his attention and concentration as well as his short- and long-term memory and comprehension of narrative discourse (meaningful, personally relevant stories in short segments in conversation with partners sensitive to his attention and memory problems). It is also recommended that J.D. be retested prior to discharge in order to monitor his recovery and develop a treatment plan.

Retesting of the PTBI

From the time of initial (prior) testing on June 3, 2009, J.D. received occupational, physical, and speech therapy on a daily basis (excluding weekends) while he was an inpatient on the pediatric rehabilitation program. He is currently receiving these therapies as an outpatient 2–3 times per week. On October 4, 2009, the PTBI was re-administered to assess J.D.'s progress. The results of this retesting are reported as ability scores and performance level ratings (with prior ability scores and performance level ratings in parentheses for comparison), as follows. (*Note:* *Indicates a score that has changed by > 1 *SEM* from the prior assessment.)

1. *Orientation*: 30.0*—Low (Prior result: 7.5—Very Low)
2. *Following Commands*: 12.0*—Low (Prior result: 5.0—Very Low)
3. *Word Fluency*: 22.0*—Low (Prior result: 2.0—Very Low)
4. *What Goes Together* (vocabulary relationships): 84.0*—High (Prior result: 22.5—Very Low)
5. *Digit Span*: 69.0*—High (Prior result: 82.5—High)
6. *Naming*: 12.5*—High (Prior result: 4.0—Very Low)
7. *Story Retelling—Immediate*: 0—Very Low (Prior result: 0—Very Low)
8. *Yes/No/Maybe* (language comprehension): 22.0*—Moderate (Prior result: 1—Very Low)
9. *Picture Recall*: 16.0*—Very Low (Prior result: 5.0—Very Low)
10. *Story Retelling—Delayed*: 0—Very Low (Prior result: 0—Very Low)
11. *Overall performance rating*: Low–Moderate (with scores in the Very Low, Low, Moderate, and High ranges)

Overall, J.D. has shown significant improvement in Orientation, Following Commands, Word Fluency, What Goes Together, Naming, and Yes/No/Maybe. He continues to have great difficulty with immediate and delayed story retelling and Picture Recall. It is recommended that J.D. continue with his outpatient therapies and be retested on at least a quarterly basis in order to monitor his recovery and to develop appropriate treatment plans. Therapy at this time should focus on improving his attention and concentration and providing him with functional listening and reading comprehension activities (meaningful texts with opportunities to discuss in a non-testlike manner). It also is recommended that J.D. have a full neuropsychological evaluation to assist in plans for school reentry and appropriate classroom accommodations (e.g., extra help, breaks, note taking).

LONGER SUMMARY

Description of the PTBI

The Pediatric Test of Brain Injury (PTBI) is a test that assesses neurocognitive and language abilities of children recovering from brain injury. The test is criterion referenced and provides cut-off scores for each subtest that can be used to describe age-related ability scores, confidence intervals, and performance category severity ratings (very low, low, moderate, and high) for categorizing how the child is functioning at a particular point in the recovery process. The PTBI also can be used for retesting, allowing comparison of scores and performance categories to gauge changes in the child's abilities.

Summary of the Results for J.D. One Month Post Onset

The results of the PTBI administered to J.D. when he was tested first at 1 month post onset yielded the following ability scores and performance level ratings:

1. *Orientation*: 7.5—Very Low
2. *Following Commands*: 5.0—Very Low
3. *Word Fluency*: 2.0—Very Low
4. *What Goes Together* (vocabulary relationships): 22.5—Very Low
5. *Digit Span*: 82.5—High
6. *Naming*: 4.0—Very Low
7. *Story Retelling—Immediate*: 0—Very Low
8. *Yes/No/Maybe* (language comprehension): 1.0—Very Low
9. *Picture Recall*: 5.0—Very Low
10. *Story Retelling—Delayed*: 0—Very Low
11. *Overall performance rating*: Very Low (except for Digit Span)

These results show the more immediate impact of J.D.'s head injury on his cognitive-linguistic functioning, which is summarized as Very Low at this early point. The testing time was 36 minutes, and J.D. scored in the Very Low range on 9 of the 10 subtests. On the Orientation Task, he was able to give his name, age, and grade (using self-correction to change 9th to 10th grade), but he could not answer any other questions about time or place and demonstrated perseveration in his attempts.

J.D. had particular difficulty on tasks that measured sentence and discourse-level comprehension ability and on following commands that most school-age children can follow without difficulty. An exception to his performance on other tasks was J.D.'s superior ability to repeat digits (Digit Span), which placed him in the High performance category. On this task, he earned the highest possible score. In contrast, J.D. was unable to remember language or picture content from tasks that required higher level cognitive-linguistic processing. He could not recall any content from a story he heard either immediately or later, and he made up (confabulated) one detail that was not in the story. He also was unable to show comprehension of discourse in the Yes/No/Maybe task, becoming upset (showing some awareness of his deficits), so the clinical decision was made to discontinue this task.

At this early point in his recovery, J.D. showed difficulty naming even simple body parts and in generating words to complete a timed Word Fluency task. He could not generate any names of animals, simply repeating the word *animals*, but did generate two words beginning with M (*mammals* and *man*). He scored slightly higher on the What Goes Together vocabulary relationships task (the upper end of the confidence interval on this subtest would put him in the Low performance category). J.D. was able to pick two different pairs of words that go together on 5 of the 7 items, but he was not able to provide reasons that earned credit for any of the pairs he selected. He said "I can't remember," "I don't know," and "I'm not sure" on 7 of 14 attempts. He did attempt a few responses that were somewhat relevant but could not receive credit for showing core relationships (e.g., nose and smell are "both on the face" [scores 0]).

J.D. will need rehabilitation to help him regain the skills needed for processing complex academic language to enable him to return to school. His rehabilitation professionals might use curricular materials from J.D.'s school to help him develop strategies for comprehending and recalling short segments of meaningful text, as well as to be able to read brief, positive social messages from his peers, or talk about personally relevant stories from home. At this point, however, J.D. is still in early stages of recovery and is not fully oriented.

All in all, PTBI testing indicates that he is likely to have great difficulty with the many competing demands of school.

Summary of Retest Results in Comparison to Earlier Results

The PTBI was re-administered to J.D. at 5 months post onset (4 months after he was first tested). By comparing his scores on the second administration to the first, it is possible to estimate J.D.'s recovery. Any retest score that is at least 1 standard error of measurement (*SEM*) (using age-appropriate values for each subtest from Appendix B) higher than the prior test score can be interpreted as representing improvement. These values are included in the list below to facilitate interpretation. (*Note*: *Indicates a score that is > 1 *SEM* higher than the prior test score.)

1. *Orientation*: 30.0*—Low (Prior result: 7.5—Very Low [0 *SEM*])
2. *Following Commands*: 12.0*—Low (Prior result: 5.0—Very Low [0 *SEM*])
3. *Word Fluency*: 22.0*—Low (Prior result: 2.0—Very Low [6 *SEM*])
4. *What Goes Together* (vocabulary relationships): 84.0*—High (Prior result: 22.5—Very Low [13 *SEM*])
5. *Digit Span*: 69.0—High (Prior result: 82.5—High [10 *SEM*])
6. *Naming*: 12.5*—High (Prior result: 4.0—Very Low [0 *SEM*])
7. *Story Retelling—Immediate*: 0—Very Low (Prior result: 0—Very Low [13 *SEM*])
8. *Yes/No/Maybe* (language comprehension): 22.0*—Moderate (Prior result: 1—Very Low [3 *SEM*])
9. *Picture Recall*: 16.0*—Very Low (Prior result: 5.0—Very Low [2 *SEM*])
10. *Story Retelling—Delayed*: 0—Very Low (Prior result: 0—Very Low [7 *SEM*])
11. *Overall performance rating*: Low–Moderate (with scores in the Very Low, Low, Moderate, and High ranges).

The retest administration of the PTBI shows that J.D. has made significant improvement in 6 of 9 subtest scores that were in the Very Low range when they were first tested. He moved from performing at Very Low to Low levels on the Orientation, answering all orientation questions correctly except for state and day of the week. He also improved from Very Low to Low on Following Commands, following all commands correctly, except for those that included the syntactic elements ("and then" and "before"). On the retest, J.D. was able to name all items on the Naming subtest, moving from Very Low to High performance on this constrained task.

J.D. also increased his performance from Very Low to Low on Word Fluency (naming 16 animals and 6 words that began with *M*); from Very Low to Moderate on Yes/No/Maybe (this time being able to complete all items without distress); and from Very Low to High on What Goes Together (this time being able to give acceptable reasons for all but 3 of 14 items). He maintained his High performance on the Digit Span task.

The one area that did not improve was the immediate and delayed recall of story components for Story Retelling. J.D. made several confabulatory comments about the story of going to a concert, for example "country music," which was not in the original story. He also missed the main problem of the narrative, which involved two friends making promises to their parents and then getting rained out of the concert. This level of comprehension difficulty needs to be addressed before J.D. can benefit from the academic discourse of school. The fact that he was able to respond appropriately to 12 out of 19 Yes/No/Maybe questions when the text remained, and to show none of the perseveration or distress that he showed at 1 month post onset, suggests that he has made significant improvement in processing complex sentence- and discourse-level discourse when memory requirements are greatly reduced. Although his Picture Recall score remained in the Very Low category, his inclusion of a hat and shoes led to an increase from a score of 5.0 to 16.0, which exceeds the *SEM* of 2, representing a significant improvement.

A transition team should begin planning activities that will facilitate J.D.'s continued recovery and possible return to school. It is a positive sign that he has made significant recovery in so many areas, but his remaining problems are significant and would present difficulties in attempting to process the language of the classroom. In particular, J.D.'s comprehension skills and strategies for facilitating recall (e.g., through discussion of short segments of text and revisualization of key components of meaningful graphic material) should be targeted in curriculum-related rehabilitation activities, and then reassessed.

Pediatric Test of Brain Injury™ (PTBI™) TEST FORM

Gillian Hotz, Nancy Helm-Estabrooks,
Nickola Wolf Nelson, and Elena Plante

PTBI™

CHILD'S INFORMATION

Child's name: J.D.
Case/medical record ID number: 472967
Child's city/state: Miami, Florida
Child's school: Everglades High School
Child's grade: 10th
Child's gender: ___ female ✓ male
Language(s) spoken: ✓ English ___ Spanish
___ Other:
Classroom performance (prior to injury):
___ below average ✓ average ___ above average
Handedness: ✓ right ___ left ___ ambidextrous
Any hand restrictions due to injury:
Any speaking restrictions due to injury (e.g. intubation):

	Year	Month	Day		Year	Month	Day
Date tested	2009	6	3	Date tested	2009	~~6~~ 5	~~3~~ 33
Date of birth	1995	5	1	Date of injury/onset	2009	5	5
Chronological age	14	1	2	Time post-injury/onset	0	0	28

Note: Subtract date of birth from date tested to get chronological age. Subtract date of onset/injury from date tested to get time post-injury/onset.

TESTING INFORMATION

Examiner's name: J.S.
Facility: West Rehabilitation Center

MEDICAL HISTORY

Primary diagnosis: TBI
Mechanism of injury: Mini motor bike (without helmet)
GCS[1] on admission: 3
GCS[1] at PTBI testing: N/A
RLAS[2] at PTBI testing: VI
CT/MRI results: Small left subdural hematoma, left frontal and temporal contusions with mass effect and cerebral edema
Surgical procedures: Frontal-parietal craniotomy for decompression
Current medications: N/A

Previous head injury: ___ yes ✓ no
Other prior problems (specify):

[1]*Glasgow Coma Scale* [2]*Rancho Los Amigos Scale*

NOTE: *If the PTBI is administered in two sessions, they must be* ***on the same day.*** *The first session must end after Subtest 5; the second session begins with Subtest 6.*

Testing time: Session 1 ______ Session 2 ______
Total testing time: 36 min.

SUMMARY SCORING CHART	Ability Score (from Test Form)	Performance Category (from Appendix A)	*SEM*	Confidence Interval	Previous Test Results
Constrained Skills		**VL** = Very Low **L** = Low **M** = Moderate **H** = High	Standard error of measurement (from Appendix B)	Add and subtract *SEM* from Ability Score	Date: ______ Ability Score Perf. Category
1. Orientation	7.5	☑ VL ☐ L ☐ M ☐ H	0	7.5 to 7.5	
2. Following Commands	5.0	☑ VL ☐ L ☐ M ☐ H	0	5.0 to 5.0	
6. Naming	4.0	☑ VL ☐ L ☐ M ☐ H	0	4.0 to 4.0	
Unconstrained Skills					
3. Word Fluency	2.0	☑ VL ☐ L ☐ M ☐ H	6	0 to 8.0	
4. What Goes Together	22.5	☑ VL ☐ L ☐ M ☐ H	13	9.5 to 35.5	
5. Digit Span	82.5	☐ VL ☐ L ☐ M ☑ H	10	72.5 to 92.5	
7. Story Retelling—Immediate	0	☑ VL ☐ L ☐ M ☐ H	13	0 to 13.0	
8. Yes/No/Maybe	1.0	☑ VL ☐ L ☐ M ☐ H	3	0 to 4.0	
9. Picture Recall	5.0	☑ VL ☐ L ☐ M ☐ H	2	3.0 to 7.0	
10. Story Retelling—Delayed	0	☑ VL ☐ L ☐ M ☐ H	7	0 to 7.0	

SUMMARY OF OVERALL PERFORMANCE: Very Low

 1

Figure 7.1. First PTBI administration for J.D.

SUBTEST 1: ORIENTATION

Materials	Test Form
Instructions	Say, ***"First, I need to find out some things about you."*** Record the child's responses verbatim. *Probe:* For last name and month, day, and year, as necessary *Note:* If the child cannot speak, accept written responses on a separate sheet. Attach written responses to Test Form.
Discontinue Rule	None
Repetition	If the child asks or does not respond within 10 seconds, each item may be repeated once.
Scoring	• Cross out ability score for any incorrect item; circle ability score for each correct item. • Add scores for correct items to compute total ability score.

Item	Question/Response	Ability Score
1	***What is your full name?*** (Child must say both first and last name. If child does not say last name on first trial, **probe** for last name.)	(0.5)
2	***How old are you?*** 14	(1.5)
3a	***When is your birthday?*** (For incomplete responses, **probe** for month, day, and year.) Month November	~~2.0~~
3b	Day 14	~~2.0~~
3c	Year 1995	(3.5)
4	***What grade are you in?*** 9th, no 10th (SC) (If summer, accept either completed or upcoming grade.)	(2.0)
5	***What school do you go to?*** New Harmony	~~3.0~~
6	***What city or town do you live in?*** Harmony (If rural address, accept nearest town.)	~~4.0~~
7	***What state/province do you live in?*** November (P)	~~3.5~~
8	***What is <u>this</u> place?*** IDK (Accept "hospital," "clinic," "school," "home," and so forth.)	~~3.5~~
9	***What day of the week is it today?*** Wednesday (P)	~~4.5~~
10	***What month is it?*** Wednesday (P)	~~4.0~~
11	***What year is it?*** November (P)	~~4.0~~

Time to administer: 4 min. **TOTAL ORIENTATION ABILITY SCORE** 7.5 / 38.0

Behavioral observations: (Abbreviations may be used next to items where they apply.)

___ Repetition of instructions (Rep)	✓ Perseveration (P)	___ No response (NR)
___ Attention reminder required (Attn)	___ Delayed response (5+ sec) (DR)	✓ I don't know (IDK)
___ Prompt to reestablish set (Prompt)	___ Unintelligible response (UnR)	✓ Self-correction (SC)

Additional qualitative/behavioral observations:

Highly perseverative. Appears disoriented to place and time, but perseveration may be partially blocking correct responding. Probe orientation informally following formal test completion.

Notes for examiners on Orientation: Orientation to person, place, and date is a key component of any examination of individuals with brain injury. By recording exact responses, you can look for behaviors, such as perseveration of earlier responses and patterns such as disorientation to time but not person or place. Individuals may have response difficulties secondary to word retrieval and production.

 3

Note: Page 2, which contains administration reminders, is excluded from this case example.

SUBTEST 2: FOLLOWING COMMANDS

Materials	Test Form
Instructions	Say, ***"Okay, now I want you to do some things without talking. Wait until I finish telling you what to do before you start. Here's one for practice."*** *Practice item:* ***"Close your eyes."*** (If the child's eyes stay shut, say, ***"Okay, now open them."***) Record deviations from each required (underlined) component. The child must demonstrate all required components in the sequence specified to receive credit.
Discontinue Rule	None
Repetition	If the child asks or does not respond within 10 seconds, each command may be repeated once.
Scoring	• Cross out ability score for any item not completely correct; circle ability score for each correct item. • Add scores for correct items to compute total ability score.

Item	Command/Response		Ability Score
1	***Where's your knee?***		(0.5)
2	***Make a fist.***		(1.5)
3	***Stick out ✓your tongue and then point to the door.***	Only tongue (Rep)	~~1.5~~
4	***Before you point to ✓the floor, ✓point to your foot.***	Pointed to the floor, then to foot.	~~1.5~~
5	***After you look at the ceiling, touch your heart.***	NR	~~1.5~~
6	***With your thumb, touch your stomach.***	Pointed to floor	~~2.5~~
7	***Look to the left and then to the right.***	OK	(3.0)
8	***Point to the light after you shake your head.***	(Rep) Repeats but no gesture	~~3.0~~

Time to administer: 3 min. **TOTAL FOLLOWING COMMANDS ABILITY SCORE** 5.0 / 15.0

Behavioral observations: (Abbreviations may be used next to items where they apply.)

✓ Repetition of instructions (Rep)	✓ Perseveration (P)	✓ No response (NR)
___ Attention reminder required (Attn)	___ Delayed response (5+ sec) (DR)	___ I don't know (IDK)
___ Prompt to reestablish set (Prompt)	___ Unintelligible response (UnR)	___ Self-correction (SC)

Additional qualitative/behavioral observations:

Perseverative behavior is both verbal (see Subtest 1) and nonverbal. Make nursing staff aware of difficulty following commands,

Notes for examiners on Following Commands: The ability to accurately follow commands is crucial for both rehabilitation and educational programs. Although examiners often assume that level of difficulty can be accounted for simply by length, item response theory analysis for this test indicated otherwise (as reflected in the scoring system). Record examinees' exact responses so you can look for behavioral patterns such as perseveration (e.g., pointing again to a particular object) and sequencing problems.

SUBTEST 3: WORD FLUENCY

3A. Semantic: Animals

Materials Test Form, Stimulus Book (page 1), watch with second hand or stopwatch

Instructions **This subtest is timed.** 60 seconds is allowed for each part.

Show the printed word ***ANIMALS*** to the child. Leave the stimulus page open for the duration of the task.

Say, ***"I want you to name as many animals as you can in 1 minute. Can you think of an animal?"***

- If the child names an animal, say, ***"Good. Name as many animals as you can. Start now."*** (Start timing and write words child says in the box for the appropriate time interval.)
- If the child stops before the minute is up, prompt, ***"Keep going. You have more time."***
- Only prompt once, but keep timing until the 60 seconds is up.

Discontinue Rule None

Repetition If the child asks or does not respond within 10 seconds, repeat the directions once.

Scoring

- Count each correct new animal named.
- Any animal or category counts (e.g., mammals, insects, birds, dinosaurs).
- Count semantic variants (e.g., *sow* and *pig* count as 2; *African elephant* and *Indian elephant* count as 2; but *baby elephant* and *big elephant* count as 1).
- Diminutive or plural forms of the same word count as 1 (e.g., *dog* and *doggie*; *cat* and *cats*).
- Do not count any word that is not an animal, is perseverated (mark P), or is a nonword.
- Do not penalize dysarthria (e.g., *agillator)* or recognizable mispronunciations (e.g., *elevant).*
- Score 1 point for each acceptable response.

0–15 seconds	16–30 seconds	31–45 seconds	45–60 seconds
"animals"	"animals"		

Animal Fluency Score 0

3B. Phonemic: *M* words

Materials	Test Form, Stimulus Book (page 2)
Instructions	Show the printed letter ***M*** to the child and leave the stimulus page open for the duration of the task. Say, ***"I want you to name as many words beginning with the letter* M *as you can in 1 minute. The letter* M *says /mmmm/. Can you think of a word starting with the letter* M?"** • If the child names a word beginning with *M,* say, ***"Good. Name as many* M *words as you can. Start now."*** (Start timing and write words child says in the box for the appropriate time interval.) • If the child stops before the minute is up, prompt him or her by saying, ***"Keep going. You have more time."*** • Only prompt once, but keep timing until the 60 seconds is up.
Discontinue Rule	None
Repetition	If the child asks or does not respond within 10 seconds, repeat the directions once.
Scoring	• Count each correct new *M* word produced. • Count proper names. • Count each derivative form (e.g., *mom, mommy,* and *mother* count as 3) but not inflected forms such as plurals (*mom* and *moms* count as 1) or inflected verb forms (*make* and *making* count as 1). • Do not count any word that is not an *M* word, is perseverated (mark P), or is a nonword. • Do not penalize dysarthria or recognizable mispronunciations. • Score 1 point for each acceptable response. • Compute total ability score by adding scores for both parts of the subtest.

0–15 seconds	16–30 seconds	31–45 seconds	45–60 seconds
mammals		man	man (P)

***M* Fluency Score** 2

Animal Fluency Score 0

TOTAL WORD FLUENCY SCORE 2

Behavioral observations: (Abbreviations may be used next to items where they apply.)

___ Repetition of instructions (Rep)	✓ Perseveration (P)	___ No response (NR)
___ Attention reminder required (Attn)	___ Delayed response (5+ sec) (DR)	___ I don't know (IDK)
___ Prompt to reestablish set (Prompt)	___ Unintelligible response (UnR)	___ Self-correction (SC)

Additional qualitative/behavioral observations:

Appeared "in set" for tasks but unable to generate any animal name and may have been prompted to say "mammals" for "m" words by animal task.

Notes for examiners on Word Fluency: Word Fluency calls on multiple cognitive-linguistic skills involved in conducting an organized mental search by category so this task is a sensitive measure of brain function. Review recorded responses for qualitative observations of performance. Positive executive behaviors include the use of subcategories of animals to aid word retrieval. Look also for negative behaviors, such as perseveration (repetition of an earlier response), as this behavior is associated with brain dysfunction. By entering responses according to time intervals, you can see whether there is consistent recall across the intervals, a warm-up effect, or quick exhaustion of the mental search. Other negative behaviors include "loss-of-set" (failure to stay on task) and partial "stuck-in-set" (e.g., naming only animals that begin with the letter *M*).

SUBTEST 4: WHAT GOES TOGETHER

Materials Test Form, Stimulus Book (pages 3–10)

Instructions *Practice item:* Begin by training the child to do this task. Open the Stimulus Book to page 3 and say, ***"Here are three words. Let's read them together."*** (Reading in unison is allowed but not required.) ***"dog–cat–bone"***

Say, **"Tell me two words that go together."**
- Circle the child's responses in the lines provided.
- The order of the child's response does not matter.

Then ask, ***"Why?"***

Probing for the practice item: If the response to the question ***"Why?"*** on the practice item is not a good/primary/dominant response, say, ***"Can you think of a better reason to put dog and cat*** [or dog and bone] ***together?"*** If the child does not say, "both are animals," or another appropriate answer, probe, ***"Do you think that they are both animals? How about that for a reason?"***

Test items: Proceed to the test items.
Say, ***"Now you will put other words together."*** Read the words aloud. Then say, ***"What two are you putting together?"*** Then ask, ***"Why?"*** Record responses verbatim.

Then say, ***"What other two are you putting together?"*** and ***"Why?"***

Do not probe for more elaborate answers within the test items. Just ask for pairings and rationales.

Note: If the child is not able to speak but can write, permit written responses.

Discontinue Rule Discontinue testing only if the child does not respond to the practice item (all parts) or gets no credit for parts a, b, c, and d for 3 consecutive items. Cross out scores for all remaining items.

Repetition None

Scoring
- Circle the responses the child gives.
- Circle the child's reason or write in a reason that is not listed.
- Both word pairs must be correct to receive word-pair credit in column on right.
- Reasons *why* are scored separately.
- Do not credit reason for any incorrect word pair.
- Cross out ability score for any incorrect item and any items past point of discontinuation; circle ability score for each correct item.
- Add subtotals for each column.
- Compute total ability score by adding the column subscores.

Practice

a **dog** — **cat** — bone
b ***Why?*** IDK
both animals, both pets (**not**—dogs chase cats [not core meaning])

c **dog** — cat — **bone**
d ***Why?*** Dog is inside the bones
dogs like / eat / bury / chew bones

Item	Item Content/Responses	Ability Score	Item	Item Content/Responses	Ability Score
1a	**red** — apple — **blue**		1c	**red** — **apple** — blue	0.5
1b	***Why?*** NR IDK both colors	~~6.0~~	1d	***Why?*** Can't remember apple is / can be red	~~6.0~~
2a	**knife** — **fork** — saw		2c	**knife** — fork — **saw**	~~5.0~~
2b	***Why?*** Can't remember things you eat with, utensils, silverware	~~2.5~~	2d	***Why?*** They might both sharp, used to cut	~~3.5~~
3a	**car** — water — **boat**		3c	car — **water** — **boat**	6.0
3b	***Why?*** The boat helps the car transportation, take you places, go in them / drive them, have motors	~~5.0~~	3d	***Why?*** Boat is in the same boat goes in / moves in / across water	~~6.0~~
4a	**mother** — **father** — daughter		4c	**mother** — father — **daughter**	5.0
4b	***Why?*** Family married, parents, takes two to make a daughter	~~4.5~~	4d	***Why?*** IDK females, girls, women, daughter comes from mother	~~2.5~~

Item	Item Content/Responses	Ability Score	Item	Item Content/Responses	Ability Score
5a	(taste) – nose – (smell)		5c	taste – (nose) – (smell)	(6.0)
5b	***Why?*** Each spot both senses [**not**—you can smell and taste food]	~~4.0~~	5d	***Why?*** Both on face smell with nose, use nose to smell	~~1.5~~

Item	Item Content/Responses	Ability Score	Item	Item Content/Responses	Ability Score
6a	painter – (elevator) – (ladder)		6c	(painter) – elevator – (ladder)	(5.0)
6b	***Why?*** The ladder holds them up use to go up and down / reach high places [**not**—go up only]	~~5.0~~	6d	***Why?*** I'm not sure painter uses / stands on ladder	~~5.5~~

Item	Item Content/Responses	Ability Score	Item	Item Content/Responses	Ability Score
7a	(bat) – (eagle) – owl		7c	(bat) – eagle – (owl)	~~6.0~~
7b	***Why?*** IDK both birds, have feathers	~~7.5~~	7d	***Why?*** I'm not sure nocturnal, up at night	~~7.5~~

Time to administer: 5 min. **Subtotal Score 1** 0 / 34.5

Subtotal Score 2 22.5 / 66.0

Subtotal Score 1 0 / 34.5

TOTAL WHAT GOES TOGETHER ABILTY SCORE 22.5 / 100.5

Behavioral observations: (Abbreviations may be used next to items where they apply.)

___ Repetition of instructions (Rep)	___ Perseveration (P)	✓ No response (NR)
___ Attention reminder required (Attn)	___ Delayed response (5+ sec) (DR)	___ I don't know (IDK)
___ Prompt to reestablish set (Prompt)	___ Unintelligible response (UnR)	___ Self-correction (SC)

Additional qualitative/behavioral observations:

Fairly good ability to pair items but almost incapable of generating rationales other than a few rather concrete associations.

Notes for examiners on What Goes Together: What Goes Together is a test of semantic/conceptual knowledge, categorical awareness, and mental flexibility. In addition to quantitative scoring of this task, you should write any nonallowed responses for qualitative information. Look for the following types of no-credit responses to "Why?": personalization (e.g., *"Because I have a mother and father")*, perseverative thought processes (e.g., *"A painter paints the ladder. A painter paints the elevator")*, emotional coloring (e.g., *"You kill with a knife and saw", "You kill an owl with a bat")*, generalizations (e.g., *"They're the same thing")*, and total failure to see a relationship (e.g., *"I don't know why")*.

SUBTEST 5: DIGIT SPAN

Materials Test Form

Instructions Say, ***"I am going to say some numbers. Listen to the numbers, and when I finish, you say them back to me exactly the same way. Wait until I stop saying numbers before you begin."***

- Present numbers at the rate of 1 per second with even stress and prosody.
- Do not chunk numbers.
- No written responses are permitted on this subtest.

Discontinue Rule Discontinue if the child fails both sequences for any item and cross out scores for remaining items.

Repetition Not allowed

Scoring
- Cross out ability score for any incorrect item or for all items following discontinuation; circle ability score for each correct item.
- Add scores for correct items to compute total ability score.

Item	Stimuli/Responses	Ability Score	Item	Stimuli/Responses	Ability Score
1a	✓ ✓ *7 – 3*	(0.5)	1b	✓ ✓ *5 – 9*	(0.5)
2a	✓ ✓ ✓ *5 – 8 – 2*	(0.5)	2b	✓ ✓ ✓ *4 – 1 – 8*	(1.0)
3a	✓ ✓ ✓ ✓ *6 – 4 – 9 – 3*	(4.0)	3b	✓ ✓ ✓ ✓ *8 – 2 – 5 – 1*	(5.0)
4a	✓ ✓ ✓ ✓ ✓ *7 – 5 – 1 – 4 – 9*	(9.5)	4b	✓ ✓ ✓ ✓ ✓ *3 – 8 – 1 – 7 – 2*	(10.0)
5a	✓ ✓ ✓ ✓ ✓ ✓ *9 – 2 – 5 – 8 – 1 – 4*	(11.5)	5b	✓ ✓ ✓ ✓ ✓ ✓ *2 – 5 – 9 – 6 – 3 – 8*	(12.5)
6a	✓ ✓ ✓ ✓ ✓ ✓ ✓ *1 – 7 – 3 – 8 – 6 – 2 – 9*	(13.5)	6b	✓ ✓ ✓ ✓ ✓ ✓ ✓ *7 – 2 – 5 – 8 – 1 – 9 – 4*	(14.0)

Time to administer: 2 min. **Subtotal Score 1** 39.5 / 39.5

Subtotal Score 2 43.0 / 43.0

Subtotal Score 1 39.5 / 39.5

TOTAL DIGIT SPAN ABILITY SCORE 82.5 / 82.5

Behavioral observations: (Abbreviations may be used next to items where they apply.)

___ Repetition of instructions (Rep)	___ Perseveration (P)	___ No response (NR)
___ Attention reminder required (Attn)	___ Delayed response (5+ sec) (DR)	___ I don't know (IDK)
___ Prompt to reestablish set (Prompt)	___ Unintelligible response (UnR)	___ Self-correction (SC)

Additional qualitative/behavioral observations:

Astonishing ability to repeat digits (up to 7 numbers) in view of performance on foregoing tasks. Very immediate memory without processing demands is excellent.

Notes for examiners on Digit Span: Digit Span is primarily a test of attention and immediate memory. In the early phase of recovery, Digit Span performance may be below normal range but then recover independently of tasks with higher level cognitive demands. You can examine qualitative patterns by writing the numbers as spoken by examinees. Look for patterns such as repeating correct numbers in the wrong order, remembering only first numbers (primacy) or last numbers (recency) in longer strings, substituting overlearned sequences (e.g., 3, 4, 5), and perseverating on numbers from earlier responses. Remember that this task requires verbal production of exact words and examinees are not allowed to write responses; therefore, it may not be a valid task for individuals who cannot speak.

NOTE: If you are administering this test in two sessions, end the first testing session here.

NOTE: *If you are administering this test in two sessions, start the second testing session here.*

SUBTEST 6: NAMING

Materials	Test Form, Stimulus Book (page 11)
Instructions	Open the Stimulus Book to page 11 and show the child the picture of the boy on his skateboard. • Ask the child the question for each item in the table below while pointing to the precise location of the target item. • If the child starts to elaborate, say, ***"Just give me one word."*** Record each response verbatim. If the child names an adjacent item, prompt, ***"No, this part."*** DO NOT tell the child to remember the picture for later
Discontinue Rule	None
Repetition	Repeat the question one time if the child does not respond within 10 seconds.
Scoring	• Cross out ability score for any incorrect item; circle ability score for each correct item. • Add scores for correct items to compute total ability score. • Do not penalize dysarthria or recognizable mispronunciations (e.g., *eblow*).

Item	Question	Target Item/Response	Ability Score
1	***What do you call these things?*** (If child names "trucks," [part of a skateboard], say, ***"No, this part,"*** and point again, specifically to wheels)	Wheels Ladder (P) (see Subtest 4)	~~0.5~~
2	***What do you call these things?*** (If child names "laces" [or other part], say, ***"No, the whole thing."***)	Boots / (Shoes)	(0.5)
3	***What do you call this thing?***	Star New Harmony (P) (see Subtest 1)	~~0.5~~
4	***What do you call this thing?***	(Chain) / ID tags / Dog tags / Necklace	(1.5)
5	***What do you call this thing?***	Band-Aid A leaf (VP)	~~2.0~~
6	***What do you call this part of his body?***	(Chin)	(2.0)
7	***And this part of his body?***	Elbow Chin (P)	~~2.5~~
8	***And this part?*** (If child names "eye" [or other part], say, ***"No, this part."***)	Eyebrow Chin (P)	~~3.0~~

Time to administer: 4 min. **TOTAL NAMING ABILITY SCORE** 4.0 / 12.5

Behavioral observations: (Abbreviations may be used next to items where they apply.)

___ Repetition of instructions (Rep)	✓ Perseveration (P)	___ No response (NR)
___ Attention reminder required (Attn)	___ Delayed response (5+ sec) (DR)	___ I don't know (IDK)
___ Prompt to reestablish set (Prompt)	___ Unintelligible response (UnR)	___ Self-correction (SC)

Additional qualitative/behavioral observations:

Performance plagued by perseverative responses and (notably) one visuoperceptual error.

Notes for examiners on Naming: Naming deficits are a key symptom of aphasia, and even delayed retrieval may be a sign of mild anomia. By recording an examinee's exact responses, you can identify error types such as semantic paraphasias (e.g., "ankle" for *elbow*), phonemic paraphasias (e.g., "eyetrow" for *eyebrow*), and circumlocutions (e.g., "put it around your neck" for *necklace/chain*), as well as perseverations. Look also for verbosity (elaboration rather than naming the item). In such cases, say, ***"Just give me one word."*** When misnaming occurs, try to identify the mechanism(s) for the error (e.g., language problem, visual acuity, visual perceptual deficits). In addition to testing naming ability, this subtest has a secondary purpose, which is to draw the examinee's attention to key elements of the picture for later recall (Subtest 9: Picture Recall). If the child comments on the danger of the skateboarder wearing a hat rather than a helmet, say, ***"You're absolutely right."***

SUBTEST 7: STORY RETELLING—IMMEDIATE

Materials Test Form, for children in:
Grades 1–3: Read Story 1, "Bobby's Lucky Day."
Grades 4–7: Read Story 2, "Tommy the Trickster."
Grades 8–11: Read Story 3, "The Rock Concert."

Instructions Say, ***"I'm going to tell you a story. Listen carefully. I want you to repeat the whole story back to me exactly as I told it to you. I can only read it once. Are you ready?"*** Although "exactly" is in the instructions to the child, some semantically acceptable substitutions, as indicated, can receive credit.

"Okay, here is the story." Use natural inflection when reading the story.

After reading the story, say, ***"Now tell me the same story. Start now."***

Probe: If the child does not initiate the story, say, ***"What was the story about? What happened?"***

DO NOT tell the child to remember the story for later.

Discontinue Rule None

Repetition Repeat the directions one time if requested.
Prompt as indicated if the child does not begin retelling the story within 10 seconds.

Scoring
- Identify each correct story element recalled and circle corresponding ability score; cross out ability score for any omitted or incorrect item.
- Count acceptable semantic substitutions as correct.
- Do not count variations that change the meaning (e.g., "street" for *sidewalk*).
- Count pronouns as correct; but at first mention, the child must say characters' proper names (*Bobby, Tommy, Daryl, Rochelle*).
- Count elements told out of sequence as correct.
- Add scores for correct items to compute total ability score.

STORY 1 (GRADES 1–3)

Read the following story: "Bobby's Lucky Day"

"Bobby's grandmother gave him some money to buy candy. On his way to the store, the money fell out of a hole in his pocket. Bobby was really upset. But suddenly, he saw a dollar on the sidewalk in front of the store. It was Bobby's lucky day!"

Say, ***"Now tell me the same story. Start now."***

Probe: If the child does not initiate the story, say, ***"What was the story about? What happened?"***

Item	**Story Elements** (optional wording)	Ability Score	Item	**Story Elements** (optional wording)	Ability Score
1	Bobby's (must use proper name to count)	0.5	12	in his pocket	1.0
2	grandmother	2.0	13	Bobby (he)	3.0
3	gave him (Bobby)	1.5	14	(really) upset / mad	4.0
4	(some) money	1.0	15	but suddenly	5.5
5	to buy	3.0	16	he (Bobby) saw	1.5
6	candy	3.0	17	a dollar	1.0
7	on his way to	4.0	18	on the sidewalk	3.0
8	the store	3.0	19	in front of	3.0
9	(the) money	2.5	20	the store	2.5
10	fell out of	1.5	21	Bobby's (his)	1.5
11	a hole	2.0	22	lucky day	1.5

Time to administer: _____ **Subtotal Score 1** _____ / 24.0

Subtotal Score 2 _____ / 27.5

Subtotal Score 1 _____ / 24.0

TOTAL STORY RETELLING—IMMEDIATE ABILTY SCORE _____ / 51.5

STORY 3 (GRADES 8–11)

Read the following story: "The Rock Concert"

"Last spring, Daryl got two free tickets to an outdoor rock concert. So, he asked his friend Rochelle to go with him. Daryl said to his father, 'If you let me go to the concert with Rochelle and drive us there, I will take out the trash for three months.' Rochelle said to her mother, 'If you let me go to the concert with Daryl and pick us up afterwards, I promise to babysit my sister six times.' Both parents agreed. Ten minutes after the kids were dropped off, it began to pour. The concert was cancelled. The kids couldn't believe it. They would still have to keep their promises!"

Say, ***"Now tell me the same story. Start now."***

Probe: If the child does not initiate the story, say, ***"What was the story about? What happened?"***

Item	**Story Elements** (optional wording)	Ability Score	Item	**Story Elements** (optional wording)	Ability Score
1	Last spring *see below	~~4.5~~	23	months	~~2.5~~
2	Daryl got (must use proper name to count)	~~2.0~~	24	Rochelle (she) said	~~4.0~~
3	two	~~3.0~~	25	to her mother	~~4.0~~
4	free	~~4.0~~	26	if you let me go (allow me to go)	~~3.5~~
5	tickets to	~~1.5~~	27	and pick us up afterwards	~~1.0~~
6	outdoor	~~5.0~~	28	I promise	~~2.5~~
7	rock	~~2.5~~	29	to babysit	~~2.5~~
8	concert	~~0.5~~	30	my sister	~~5.0~~
9	so he asked	~~2.5~~	31	six times	~~5.0~~
10	his friend	~~3.0~~	32	both parents	~~5.0~~
11	Rochelle (must use proper name to count)	~~3.0~~	33	agreed	~~5.0~~
12	to go	~~3.5~~	34	ten	~~4.0~~
13	with him	~~4.0~~	35	minutes	~~3.5~~
14	Daryl (he) said	~~3.0~~	36	after the kids	~~1.0~~
15	to his father	~~2.0~~	37	were dropped off	~~2.5~~
16	if you let me go	~~3.0~~	38	it began to "pour" (rain)	~~2.0~~
17	to the concert	~~3.5~~	39	the concert	~~3.0~~
18	with Rochelle (her)	~~3.5~~	40	was cancelled	~~5.5~~
19	and drive us (there) (give us a ride)	~~4.0~~	41	the kids (they)	~~2.0~~
20	I will take out	~~2.0~~	42	couldn't believe it (**not**—they were mad)	~~5.5~~
21	the trash (garbage)	~~3.0~~	43	would still have to	~~2.0~~
22	three	~~2.5~~	44	keep their promises (do their jobs)	~~2.0~~

Time to administer: 3 min. **Subtotal Score 1** 0 / 65.5

* Said, "The mothers are fighting."

Subtotal Score 2 0 / 73.0

Subtotal Score 1 0 / 65.5

TOTAL STORY RETELLING—IMMEDIATE ABILTY SCORE 0 / 138.5

Behavioral observations: (Abbreviations may be used next to items where they apply.)

___ Repetition of instructions (Rep)
___ Attention reminder required (Attn)
___ Prompt to reestablish set (Prompt)
___ Perseveration (P)
___ Delayed response (5+ sec) (DR)
___ Unintelligible response (UnR)
___ No response (NR)
___ I don't know (IDK)
___ Self-correction (SC)

Additional qualitative/behavioral observations:

Compared with Digit Span, poor story recall and probably comprehension difficulty. The "fighting" is confusing—filling in "gaps" in knowledge of story.

13

Note: Page 12 excluded because not relevant to this age range.

SUBTEST 8: YES/NO/MAYBE

Materials Test Form, Stimulus Book (pages 12–17)

Instructions Open the Stimulus Book to page 12 in front of the child.

Say, ***"Now we're going to read some very short stories together. I'll read and you follow along."*** (If the child can read aloud and wants to, let him or her do so. Do not require choral reading.)

Say, ***"Pay careful attention, because I'm going to ask you some questions after each story. Your answer can be 'yes' if you are certain the answer is 'yes,' or 'no' if you are certain the answer is 'no.' If the story doesn't clearly tell you the answer, you should say 'maybe.' Here is a practice item."***

- Do not remove the Stimulus Book; keep it in front of the child.
- Circle *Y* for "yes," *N* for "no," and *M* for "maybe" answers. Correct answers are in bold.

Note: If the child is unable to speak, write YES NO MAYBE in a vertical array on a piece of paper to allow a pointing response.

Discontinue Rule Discontinue testing if the child cannot get into set for the task after coaching on the practice story or if the child misses all items on two consecutive stories.

Repetition Only allowed during the practice story

Scoring
- Score self-corrections as correct only if immediate.
- Circle ability score for correct items; cross out ability score for incorrect items or items following discontinuation.
- Add subtotals for each short story.
- Compute total ability score by adding the story subscores.

Practice Story Say, ***"One morning, Susan missed the school bus. She thought she would be late for school, but her mother got her there on time."*** Say, ***"I can help you read it again if you want."***

Reread the story as often as requested, and then ask the following questions. Reinforce the correct answer for each practice question, and help the child to see the relationship if necessary.

a	***"Did Susan miss the bus?"***	**(Y)** (circled)	N	M	
b	***"Was Susan late for school?"***	Y (circled)	**(N)**	M	
c	***"Was it raining that morning?"***	Y (circled)	N	**(M)**	(P)
d	***"Did her father take her to school?"***	Y (circled)	**(N)**	M	

Short Story 1 (Turn to page 13 in the Stimulus Book. *Note:* This story has only three questions.)

The kids ran after the blue ice cream truck. It turned the corner before they could catch it.

Item	Questions	Responses	Ability Score
a	***Did the kids chase the ice cream truck?***	**(Y)** (circled) N M	0.5 (circled)
b	***Did the kids catch the truck before it turned the corner?***	Y (circled) **(N)** M	~~0.5~~
c	***Was the ice cream truck red?***	Y (circled) **(N)** M	~~0.5~~

Story 1 Ability Score 0.5 / 1.5

Short Story 2 (Turn to page 14 in the Stimulus Book.)

"What I did on my summer vacation" is the topic the teacher makes her class write about on the first day of school every year. When school started a month ago, the teacher gave her usual first writing assignment.

Item	Questions	Responses	Ability Score
a	***Did the teacher ask her class to write about their summer vacations?***	**(Y)** (circled) N M	0.5 (circled)
b	***Was the Middle East the first writing topic of the year?***	Y (circled) **(N)** M	~~3.5~~
c	***Did school start last week?***	Y (circled) **(N)** M	~~1.0~~
d	***Did all of the students take a trip on their summer vacations?***	Y (circled) N **(M)**	~~2.0~~

Discontinued when became upset.

Story 2 Ability Score 0.5 / 7.0
Story 1 Ability Score 0.5 / 1.5
Subtotal Score 1.0 / 8.5

Short Story 3 (Turn to page 15 in the Stimulus Book.) NOTE: Discontinued due to J.D. becoming upset.			
Immanuel was the first one of a small group of boys in his class who could dunk a basketball.			
Item	**Questions**	**Responses**	**Ability Score**
~~a~~	***Could Immanuel jump the highest in class?***	Y N **(M)**	~~1.0~~
~~b~~	***Could some of the other boys dunk a basketball?***	**(Y)** N M	~~2.5~~
~~c~~	***Could all of the boys in Immanuel's class dunk a basketball?***	Y **(N)** M	~~2.5~~
~~d~~	***Was Immanuel the best basketball player in his class?***	Y N **(M)**	~~2.0~~
		Story 3 Ability Score	0 / 8.0

Short Story 4 (Turn to page 16 in the Stimulus Book.)			
Mary and Todd decided they would go to the beach on Saturday even if it was a cloudy day. When they woke up on Saturday, it was sunny.			
Item	**Questions**	**Responses**	**Ability Score**
~~a~~	***Did Mary and Todd plan to go to the beach on Saturday if it was cloudy?***	**(Y)** N M	~~2.0~~
~~b~~	***Did it rain later on Saturday?***	Y N **(M)**	~~4.0~~
~~c~~	***Was it cloudy when Mary and Todd woke up on Saturday?***	Y **(N)** M	~~2.5~~
~~d~~	***Was Mary the mother of Todd?***	Y N **(M)**	~~2.0~~
		Story 4 Ability Score	0 / 10.5

Short Story 5 (Turn to page 17 in the Stimulus Book.)			
The scientists observed the insects closely over a 24-hour period, hoping to study their swarming behavior. At that point, the scientists concluded that the insects had been prevented from swarming because of the unusual atmospheric conditions.			
Item	**Questions**	**Responses**	**Ability Score**
~~a~~	***Did the insects swarm?***	Y **(N)** M	~~4.5~~
~~b~~	***Did the scientists watch the insects for a full day?***	**(Y)** N M	~~0.5~~
~~c~~	***Can atmospheric conditions influence the swarming of insects?***	**(Y)** N M	~~2.5~~
~~d~~	***Did the scientists accomplish their original goal?***	Y **(N)** M	~~4.5~~

Time to administer: 5 min.

Story 5 Ability Score	0 / 12.0
Story 4 Ability Score	0 / 10.5
Story 3 Ability Score	0 / 8.0
Subtotal from page 14	1.0 / 8.5
TOTAL YES/NO/MAYBE ABILITY SCORE	1.0 / 39.0

Behavioral observations: (Abbreviations may be used next to items where they apply.)

___ Repetition of instructions (Rep)	✓ Perseveration (P)	___ No response (NR)
___ Attention reminder required (Attn)	___ Delayed response (5+ sec) (DR)	___ I don't know (IDK)
___ Prompt to reestablish set (Prompt)	___ Unintelligible response (UnR)	___ Self-correction (SC)

Additional qualitative/behavioral observations:
Perseverative use of "yes," which by chance earned 1 point. Seemed to sense poor performance and became upset, so discontinued test after Story 2.

Notes for examiners on Yes/No/Maybe: The Yes/No/Maybe subtest was designed to test the ability to listen to/read short stories carefully enough to answer questions regarding both stated and inferred information. As such, this subtest requires several cognitive processes, including higher level language comprehension skills, attention, and mental tracking. In addition to computing the overall ability score, look for error patterns such as missing "maybe" responses or perseverating on one answer choice.

15

SUBTEST 9: PICTURE RECALL

Materials Test Form, Stimulus Book (page 11)

Instructions Say, ***"Remember the picture of the boy that I showed you a while ago?"*** If the child can't recall the picture, cue by saying, ***"The one where you named some parts of his body and other things."*** Then say, ***"Please draw that boy on this page."***

Use the last page of this Test Form.

Say, ***"Put in as many details as you can remember."***

Probe: If the child still can't remember the picture, say to the child, ***"Just draw a picture of any boy."***

When the child is finished or you see that he or she is not being productive, say, ***"Now we need your autograph. Please sign your first and last name on the bottom of your picture. Write it clearly so that anyone could read it."*** (Point to the bottom of the page.)

Probe: Okay to probe for last name if only first name is given.

Probe: If the picture is unclear or if the child is unable to draw, ask for a description, write down what the child says, and score recalled elements.

If the child cannot move to write his or her name, ask for a spelling. All letters in the name must be correct to receive credit.

Discontinue Rule If the child does not respond after 10 seconds following allowed prompting, discontinue.

Repetition If the child does not respond within 10 seconds, repeat the instructions and use the probe.

Scoring

- Circle ability score for any component recognizable in context.
- Cross out ability score for any missing component.
- All letters in name must be legible and correct for name to receive credit.
- Add subtotals for each column.
- Compute total ability score by adding the column subtotals.

Item	Picture Recall	Ability Score
1	Picture of a boy	(1.5)
2	Skateboard	~~3.0~~
3	Hat / Baseball cap	~~5.5~~
4	Boots / Shoes	~~5.5~~
5	Star	~~6.0~~
6	Chain / ID tags / Dog tags / Necklace	~~6.0~~
7	Band-Aid	~~7.0~~
8	Shorts	~~7.5~~
	Picture Recall Subtotal	1.5 / 42.0

Item	Signature	Ability Score
1	First name	(0.5)
2	Last name	(3.0)

Signature Subtotal 3.5 / 3.5

Picture Recall Subtotal 1.5 /42.0

TOTAL PICTURE RECALL ABILITY SCORE 5.0 / 45.5

Time to administer: 4 min.

Hand used: ____ L ✓ R

Behavioral observations: (Abbreviations may be used next to items where they apply.)

___ Repetition of instructions (Rep)	___ Perseveration (P)	___ No response (NR)
___ Attention reminder required (Attn)	___ Delayed response (5+ sec) (DR)	___ I don't know (IDK)
___ Prompt to reestablish set (Prompt)	___ Unintelligible response (UnR)	___ Self-correction (SC)

Additional qualitative/behavioral observations:

Micrographia—tiny figure with no recalled details. Poor delayed memory (uncued incidental).

Notes for examiners on Picture Recall: This subtest assesses incidental memory (i.e., without instruction to remember) for the picture presented in Subtest 6 and ability to depict recalled elements of that picture (through drawing, or speaking, in the case of individuals who are unable to hold a pen). The recalled components are scored, but it is important that you study the picture carefully and look for such features as micrographia (tiny drawing), proportionality, perseverative elements, unilateral neglect (drawing only half the picture), and fragmentation (refer to the *PTBI Examiner's Manual* for examples). Signatures as well as spelling can be analyzed for some of these same features.

SUBTEST 10: STORY RETELLING—DELAYED

Materials Test Form, for children in: **Grades 1–3:** Score Story 1, "Bobby's Lucky Day."
Grades 4–7: Score Story 2, "Tommy the Trickster."
Grades 8–11: Score Story 3, "The Rock Concert."

Instructions Do not reread the story. The child must recall the story from the prior experience.

Say, ***"Remember the story [title of story child heard]? Tell me the story again. Try to remember as much as you can."***

As the child retells the story, check story elements recalled correctly or record verbatim any content variations in the story produced.

Discontinue Rule None

Repetition Repeat the directions one time if requested.

Scoring

- Identify each correct story element recalled and circle corresponding ability score; cross out ability score for any omitted or incorrect item.
- Count acceptable semantic substitutions as correct.
- Do not count variations that change the meaning (e.g., "street" for *sidewalk*).
- Count pronouns as correct; but at first mention, the child must say characters' proper names (*Bobby, Tommy, Daryl, Rochelle).*
- Count elements told out of sequence as correct.
- Add scores for correct items to compute total ability score.

STORY 1 (GRADES 1–3)

Say, ***"Remember the story 'Bobby's Lucky Day'? Tell me the story again. Try to remember as much as you can"***

Item	**Story Elements** (optional wording)	Ability Score
1	Bobby's (must use proper name to count)	1.5
2	grandmother	1.5
3	gave him (Bobby)	1.5
4	(some) money	1.5
5	to buy	3.5
6	candy	3.5
7	on his way to	4.0
8	the store	3.0
9	(the) money	2.0
10	fell out of	1.5
11	a hole	2.0

Time to administer: _____ **Subtotal Score 1** _____ / 25.5

Item	**Story Elements** (optional wording)	Ability Score
12	in his pocket	1.0
13	Bobby (he)	3.5
14	(really) upset / mad	4.5
15	but suddenly	5.5
16	he (Bobby) saw	0.5
17	a dollar	0.5
18	on the sidewalk	3.0
19	in front of	3.5
20	the store	2.5
21	Bobby's (his)	2.0
22	lucky day	2.0

Subtotal Score 2 _____ / 28.5

Subtotal Score 1 _____ / 25.5

TOTAL STORY RETELLING—DELAYED ABILTY SCORE _____ / 51.5

STORY 3 (GRADES 8–11)

Say. ***Remember the story 'The Rock Concert'? Tell me the story again. Try to remember as much as you can."***

Item	**Story Elements** (optional wording)	Ability Score	Item	**Story Elements** (optional wording)	Ability Score
1	Last spring *Went to Harmony (P)*	~~4.0~~	23	months	~~2.5~~
2	Daryl got (must use proper name to count)	~~2.0~~	24	Rochelle (she) said	~~2.5~~
3	two	~~2.5~~	25	to her mother	~~1.5~~
4	free	~~4.0~~	26	if you let me go (allow me to go)	~~3.0~~
5	tickets to	~~1.0~~	27	and pick us up afterwards	~~3.0~~
6	outdoor	~~4.5~~	28	I promise	~~2.5~~
7	rock	~~1.5~~	29	to babysit	~~1.0~~
8	concert	~~0.5~~	30	my sister	~~2.5~~
9	so he asked	~~2.0~~	31	six times	~~2.5~~
10	his friend	~~2.5~~	32	both parents	~~4.0~~
11	Rochelle (must use proper name to count)	~~2.5~~	33	agreed	~~3.5~~
12	to go	~~2.5~~	34	ten	~~3.5~~
13	with him	~~3.5~~	35	minutes	~~3.5~~
14	Daryl (he) said	~~2.5~~	36	after the kids	~~3.0~~
15	to his father	~~1.5~~	37	were dropped off	~~3.0~~
16	if you let me go	~~3.0~~	38	it began to "pour" (rain)	~~1.0~~
17	to the concert	~~4.0~~	39	the concert	~~1.0~~
18	with Rochelle (her)	~~4.5~~	40	was cancelled	~~1.5~~
19	and drive us (there) (give us a ride)	~~3.0~~	41	the kids (they)	~~3.0~~
20	I will take out	~~1.5~~	42	couldn't believe it [**not**—they were mad]	~~3.5~~
21	the trash (garbage)	~~1.0~~	43	would still have to	~~1.5~~
22	three	~~2.5~~	44	keep their promises (do their jobs)	~~1.5~~

Time to administer: *4 min.* **Subtotal Score 1** *0* / 56.5

Subtotal Score 2 *0* / 54.5
Subtotal Score 1 *0* / 56.5
TOTAL STORY RETELLING—DELAYED ABILTY SCORE *0* / 111.0

Behavioral observations: (Abbreviations may be used next to items where they apply.)

___ Repetition of instructions (Rep)	✓ Perseveration (P)	___ No response (NR)
___ Attention reminder required (Attn)	___ Delayed response (5+ sec) (DR)	___ I don't know (IDK)
___ Prompt to reestablish set (Prompt)	___ Unintelligible response (UnR)	___ Self-correction (SC)

Additional qualitative/behavioral observations:

Again perseveration on "Harmony"—carried over from Subtest 1—filling in where he has no recall of story.

 19

Note: Page 18 excluded because not relevant to this age range.

SUBTEST 9: PICTURE RECALL

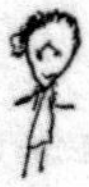

Pediatric Test of Brain Injury™ (PTBI™) TEST FORM

Gillian Hotz, Nancy Helm-Estabrooks,
Nickola Wolf Nelson, and Elena Plante

PTBI

CHILD'S INFORMATION

Child's name: J.D.

Case/medical record ID number: N/A

Child's city/state: Miami, Florida

Child's school: Everglades High School

Child's grade: 10th

Child's gender: ___ female ✓ male

Language(s) spoken: ✓ English ___ Spanish

___ Other: ___

Classroom performance (prior to injury):

___ below average ✓ average ___ above average

Handedness: ✓ right ___ left ___ ambidextrous

Any hand restrictions due to injury: ___

Any speaking restrictions due to injury (e.g. intubation): ___

	Year	Month	Day		Year	Month	Day
Date tested	2009	10	4	Date tested	2009	~~10~~ 9	~~4~~ 34
Date of birth	1995	5	1	Date of injury/onset	2009	5	5
Chronological age	14	5	3	Time post-injury/onset	0	4	29

Note: Subtract date of birth from date tested to get chronological age. Subtract date of onset/injury from date tested to get time post-injury/onset.

TESTING INFORMATION

Examiner's name: T.L.

Facility: Sunnyside Outpatient Rehabilitation Center

MEDICAL HISTORY

Primary diagnosis: TBI

Mechanism of injury: Mini motor bike (without helmet)

GCS[1] on admission: 3

GCS[1] at PTBI testing: 14

RLAS[2] at PTBI testing: VIII

CT/MRI results: Small left subdural hematoma, left frontal and temporal contusions with mass effect and cerebral edema

Surgical procedures: Frontal-parietal craniotomy for decompression

Current medications: N/A

Previous head injury: ___ yes ✓ no

Other prior problems (specify): ___

[1]Glasgow Coma Scale [2]Rancho Los Amigos Scale

***NOTE:** If the PTBI is administered in two sessions, they must be **on the same day**. The first session must end after Subtest 5; the second session begins with Subtest 6.*

Testing time: Session 1 ___ Session 2 ___

Total testing time: 40 min., 50 sec.

SUMMARY SCORING CHART	Ability Score (from Test Form)	Performance Category (from Appendix A)	SEM	Confidence Interval	Previous Test Results	
Constrained Skills		**VL** = Very Low **L** = Low **M** = Moderate **H** = High	Standard error of measurement (from Appendix B)	Add and subtract *SEM* from Ability Score	Date: 5-1-09 Ability Score	Perf. Category
1. Orientation	30.0	☐ VL ☑ L ☐ M ☐ H	0	30.0 to 30.0	7.5	VL
2. Following Commands	12.0	☐ VL ☑ L ☐ M ☐ H	0	12.0 to 12.0	5.0	VL
6. Naming	12.5	☐ VL ☐ L ☐ M ☑ H	0	12.5 to 12.5	4.0	VL
Unconstrained Skills						
3. Word Fluency	22.0	☐ VL ☑ L ☐ M ☐ H	6	16.0 to 28.0	2.0	VL
4. What Goes Together	84.0	☐ VL ☐ L ☐ M ☑ H	13	71.0 to 97.0	22.5	VL
5. Digit Span	69.0	☐ VL ☐ L ☐ M ☑ H	10	59.0 to 79.0	82.5	H
7. Story Retelling—Immediate	0	☑ VL ☐ L ☐ M ☐ H	13	0 to 13.0	0	VL
8. Yes/No/Maybe	22.0	☐ VL ☐ L ☑ M ☐ H	3	19.0 to 25.0	1.0	VL
9. Picture Recall	16.0	☑ VL ☐ L ☐ M ☐ H	2	14.0 to 18.0	5.0	VL
10. Story Retelling—Delayed	0	☑ VL ☐ L ☐ M ☐ H	7	0 to 7.0	0	VL

SUMMARY OF OVERALL PERFORMANCE: Low–Moderate

1

Figure 7.2. PTBI retest for J.D.

SUBTEST 1: ORIENTATION

Materials	Test Form
Instructions	Say, ***"First, I need to find out some things about you."*** Record the child's responses verbatim. *Probe:* For last name and month, day, and year, as necessary *Note:* If the child cannot speak, accept written responses on a separate sheet. Attach written responses to Test Form.
Discontinue Rule	None
Repetition	If the child asks or does not respond within 10 seconds, each item may be repeated once.
Scoring	• Cross out ability score for any incorrect item; circle ability score for each correct item. • Add scores for correct items to compute total ability score.

Item	Question/Response	Ability Score
1	***What is your full name?*** (Child must say both first and last name. If child does not say last name on first trial, **probe** for last name.)	(0.5)
2	***How old are you?***	(1.5)
3a	***When is your birthday?*** (For incomplete responses, **probe** for month, day, and year.) Month	(2.0)
3b	Day	(2.0)
3c	Year	(3.5)
4	***What grade are you in?*** (If summer, accept either completed or upcoming grade.)	(2.0)
5	***What school do you go to?***	(3.0)
6	***What city or town do you live in?*** (If rural address, accept nearest town.)	(4.0)
7	***What state/province do you live in?*** Miami	~~3.5~~
8	***What is <u>this</u> place?*** (Accept "hospital," "clinic," "school," "home," and so forth.)	(3.5)
9	***What day of the week is it today?*** Wednesday	~~4.5~~
10	***What month is it?***	(4.0)
11	***What year is it?***	(4.0)

Time to administer: 3 min., 20 sec. **TOTAL ORIENTATION ABILITY SCORE** 30.0 / 38.0

Behavioral observations: (Abbreviations may be used next to items where they apply.)

___ Repetition of instructions (Rep)	✓ Perseveration (P)	___ No response (NR)
___ Attention reminder required (Attn)	___ Delayed response (5+ sec) (DR)	___ I don't know (IDK)
___ Prompt to reestablish set (Prompt)	___ Unintelligible response (UnR)	___ Self-correction (SC)

Additional qualitative/behavioral observations:

Much improved on orientation and lessening of perseverative responding from Test 1.

Notes for examiners on Orientation: Orientation to person, place, and date is a key component of any examination of individuals with brain injury. By recording exact responses, you can look for behaviors, such as perseveration of earlier responses and patterns such as disorientation to time but not person or place. Individuals may have response difficulties secondary to word retrieval and production.

 3

Note: Page 2, which contains administration reminders, is excluded from this case example.

SUBTEST 2: FOLLOWING COMMANDS

Materials Test Form

Instructions Say, ***"Okay, now I want you to do some things without talking. Wait until I finish telling you what to do before you start. Here's one for practice."***

Practice item: ***"Close your eyes."*** (If the child's eyes stay shut, say, ***"Okay, now open them."***)

Record deviations from each required (underlined) component. The child must demonstrate all required components in the sequence specified to receive credit.

Discontinue Rule None

Repetition If the child asks or does not respond within 10 seconds, each command may be repeated once.

Scoring
- Cross out ability score for any item not completely correct; circle ability score for each correct item.
- Add scores for correct items to compute total ability score.

Item	Command/Response		Ability Score
1	***Where's your knee?***		(0.5)
2	***Make a fist.***		(1.5)
3	***Stick out your tongue and then point to the door.***	Stuck out tongue at door	~~1.5~~
4	***Before you point to the floor, point ✓ to your foot.***	Did not point to floor.	~~1.5~~
5	***After you look at the ceiling, touch your heart.***		(1.5)
6	***With your thumb, touch your stomach.***		(2.5)
7	***Look to the left and then to the right.***		(3.0)
8	***Point to the light after you shake your head.***		(3.0)

Time to administer: 4 min. **TOTAL FOLLOWING COMMANDS ABILITY SCORE** 12.0 / 15.0

Behavioral observations: (Abbreviations may be used next to items where they apply.)

___ Repetition of instructions (Rep)	___ Perseveration (P)	___ No response (NR)
___ Attention reminder required (Attn)	___ Delayed response (5+ sec) (DR)	___ I don't know (IDK)
___ Prompt to reestablish set (Prompt)	___ Unintelligible response (UnR)	___ Self-correction (SC)

Additional qualitative/behavioral observations:

Greatly increased accuracy from Test 1, although problems remain that may interfere with grade-level performance.

Notes for examiners on Following Commands: The ability to accurately follow commands is crucial for both rehabilitation and educational programs. Although examiners often assume that level of difficulty can be accounted for simply by length, item response theory analysis for this test indicated otherwise (as reflected in the scoring system). Record examinees' exact responses so you can look for behavioral patterns such as perseveration (e.g., pointing again to a particular object) and sequencing problems.

SUBTEST 3: WORD FLUENCY

3A. Semantic: Animals

Materials Test Form, Stimulus Book (page 1), watch with second hand or stopwatch

Instructions **This subtest is timed.** 60 seconds is allowed for each part.

Show the printed word ***ANIMALS*** to the child. Leave the stimulus page open for the duration of the task.

Say, ***"I want you to name as many animals as you can in 1 minute. Can you think of an animal?"***

- If the child names an animal, say, ***"Good. Name as many animals as you can. Start now."*** (Start timing and write words child says in the box for the appropriate time interval.)
- If the child stops before the minute is up, prompt, ***"Keep going. You have more time."***
- Only prompt once, but keep timing until the 60 seconds is up.

Discontinue Rule None

Repetition If the child asks or does not respond within 10 seconds, repeat the directions once.

Scoring
- Count each correct new animal named.
- Any animal or category counts (e.g., mammals, insects, birds, dinosaurs).
- Count semantic variants (e.g., *sow* and *pig* count as 2; *African elephant* and *Indian elephant* count as 2; but *baby elephant* and *big elephant* count as 1).
- Diminutive or plural forms of the same word count as 1 (e.g., *dog* and *doggie*; *cat* and *cats*).
- Do not count any word that is not an animal, is perseverated (mark P), or is a nonword.
- Do not penalize dysarthria (e.g., *agillator)* or recognizable mispronunciations (e.g., *elevant).*
- Score 1 point for each acceptable response.

0–15 seconds	16–30 seconds	31–45 seconds	45–60 seconds
pigs dogs cats chickens cows birds	snakes elephants tigers lions	horse cows (P) iguana	lizards rats rabbits chipmunks

Animal Fluency Score 16

3B. Phonemic: *M* words

Materials Test Form, Stimulus Book (page 2)

Instructions Show the printed letter ***M*** to the child and leave the stimulus page open for the duration of the task.

Say, ***"I want you to name as many words beginning with the letter* M *as you can in 1 minute. The letter* M *says /mmmm/. Can you think of a word starting with the letter* M?"**

- If the child names a word beginning with *M,* say, ***"Good. Name as many* M *words as you can. Start now."*** (Start timing and write words child says in the box for the appropriate time interval.)
- If the child stops before the minute is up, prompt him or her by saying, ***"Keep going. You have more time."***
- Only prompt once, but keep timing until the 60 seconds is up.

Discontinue Rule None

Repetition If the child asks or does not respond within 10 seconds, repeat the directions once.

Scoring

- Count each correct new *M* word produced.
- Count proper names.
- Count each derivative form (e.g., *mom, mommy,* and *mother* count as 3) but not inflected forms such as plurals (*mom* and *moms* count as 1) or inflected verb forms (*make* and *making* count as 1).
- Do not count any word that is not an *M* word, is perseverated (mark P), or is a nonword.
- Do not penalize dysarthria or recognizable mispronunciations.
- Score 1 point for each acceptable response.
- Compute total ability score by adding scores for both parts of the subtest.

0–15 seconds	16–30 seconds	31–45 seconds	45–60 seconds
man mother mouse	mouth Monday		more mouse (P)

***M* Fluency Score** 6

Animal Fluency Score 16

TOTAL WORD FLUENCY SCORE 22

Behavioral observations: (Abbreviations may be used next to items where they apply.)

___ Repetition of instructions (Rep)
___ Attention reminder required (Attn)
___ Prompt to reestablish set (Prompt)
✓ Perseveration (P)
___ Delayed response (5+ sec) (DR)
___ Unintelligible response (UnR)
___ No response (NR)
___ I don't know (IDK)
___ Self-correction (SC)

Additional qualitative/behavioral observations:

Impressive improvement, especially on animal fluency. Residual tendency toward perseveration—now may be linked to memory for previous responses.

Notes for examiners on Word Fluency: Word Fluency calls on multiple cognitive-linguistic skills involved in conducting an organized mental search by category so this task is a sensitive measure of brain function. Review recorded responses for qualitative observations of performance. Positive executive behaviors include the use of subcategories of animals to aid word retrieval. Look also for negative behaviors, such as perseveration (repetition of an earlier response), as this behavior is associated with brain dysfunction. By entering responses according to time intervals, you can see whether there is consistent recall across the intervals, a warm-up effect, or quick exhaustion of the mental search. Other negative behaviors include "loss-of-set" (failure to stay on task) and partial "stuck-in-set" (e.g., naming only animals that begin with the letter *M*).

SUBTEST 4: WHAT GOES TOGETHER

Materials Test Form, Stimulus Book (pages 3–10)

Instructions *Practice item:* Begin by training the child to do this task. Open the Stimulus Book to page 3 and say, ***"Here are three words. Let's read them together."*** (Reading in unison is allowed but not required.) ***"dog–cat–bone"***

Say, **"Tell me two words that go together."**

- Circle the child's responses in the lines provided.
- The order of the child's response does not matter.

Then ask, ***"Why?"***

Probing for the practice item: If the response to the question ***"Why?"*** on the practice item is not a good/primary/dominant response, say, ***"Can you think of a better reason to put dog and cat*** [or dog and bone] ***together?"*** If the child does not say, "both are animals," or another appropriate answer, probe, ***"Do you think that they are both animals? How about that for a reason?"***

Test items: Proceed to the test items.

Say, ***"Now you will put other words together."*** Read the words aloud. Then say, ***"What two are you putting together?"*** Then ask, ***"Why?"*** Record responses verbatim.

Then say, ***"What other two are you putting together?"*** and ***"Why?"***

Do not probe for more elaborate answers within the test items. Just ask for pairings and rationales.

Note: If the child is not able to speak but can write, permit written responses.

Discontinue Rule Discontinue testing only if the child does not respond to the practice item (all parts) or gets no credit for parts a, b, c, and d for 3 consecutive items. Cross out scores for all remaining items.

Repetition None

Scoring

- Circle the responses the child gives.
- Circle the child's reason or write in a reason that is not listed.
- Both word pairs must be correct to receive word-pair credit in column on right.
- Reasons *why* are scored separately.
- Do not credit reason for any incorrect word pair.
- Cross out ability score for any incorrect item and any items past point of discontinuation; circle ability score for each correct item.
- Add subtotals for each column.
- Compute total ability score by adding the column subscores.

Practice

a **dog** — **cat** — bone

b ***Why?***
both animals, both pets (**not**—dogs chase cats [not core meaning])

c **dog** — cat — **bone**

d ***Why?*** Bones inside dog
dogs like / eat / bury / chew bones

Item	Item Content/Responses	Ability Score	Item	Item Content/Responses	Ability Score
1a	**red** – apple – **blue**		1c	**red** – **apple** – blue	0.5
1b	***Why?*** both colors	6.0	1d	***Why?*** apple is / can be red	6.0
2a	**knife** – **fork** – saw		2c	**knife** – fork – **saw**	5.0
2b	***Why?*** things you eat with, utensils, silverware	2.5	2d	***Why?*** both sharp, used to cut	3.5
3a	**car** – water – **boat**		3c	car – **water** – **boat**	6.0
3b	***Why?*** Car goes somewhere transportation, take you places, go in them / drive them, have motors	~~5.0~~	3d	***Why?*** Boat goes inside water boat goes in / moves in / across water	6.0
4a	**mother** – **father** – daughter		4c	**mother** – father – **daughter**	5.0
4b	***Why?*** married, parents, takes two to make a daughter	4.5	4d	***Why?*** females, girls, women, daughter comes from mother	2.5

Item	Item Content/Responses	Ability Score	Item	Item Content/Responses	Ability Score
5a	taste – nose – smell		5c	taste – nose – smell	6.0
5b	***Why?*** Your nose smells and tastes both senses [**not**—you can smell and taste food]	~~4.0~~	5d	***Why?*** smell with nose, use nose to smell	1.5
6a	painter – elevator – ladder		6c	painter – elevator – ladder	5.0
6b	***Why?*** use to go up and down / reach high places [**not**—go up only]	5.0	6d	***Why?*** painter uses / stands on ladder	5.5
7a	bat – eagle – owl		7c	bat – eagle – owl	6.0
7b	***Why?*** both birds, have feathers	7.5	7d	***Why?*** Can fly and live in hole nocturnal, up at night	~~7.5~~

Time to administer: 5 min. **Subtotal Score 1** 25.5 / 34.5

Subtotal Score 2 58.5 / 66.0
Subtotal Score 1 25.5 / 34.5
TOTAL WHAT GOES TOGETHER ABILTY SCORE 84.0 / 100.5

Behavioral observations: (Abbreviations may be used next to items where they apply.)

___ Repetition of instructions (Rep)
___ Attention reminder required (Attn)
___ Prompt to reestablish set (Prompt)
___ Perseveration (P)
___ Delayed response (5+ sec) (DR)
___ Unintelligible response (UnR)
___ No response (NR)
___ I don't know (IDK)
___ Self-correction (SC)

Additional qualitative/behavioral observations:

Although remarkably improved, residual problem with explaining commonalities.

Notes for examiners on What Goes Together: What Goes Together is a test of semantic/conceptual knowledge, categorical awareness, and mental flexibility. In addition to quantitative scoring of this task, you should write any nonallowed responses for qualitative information. Look for the following types of no-credit responses to "Why?": personalization (e.g., *"Because I have a mother and father"*), perseverative thought processes (e.g., *"A painter paints the ladder. A painter paints the elevator"*), emotional coloring (e.g., *"You kill with a knife and saw", "You kill an owl with a bat"*), generalizations (e.g., *"They're the same thing"*), and total failure to see a relationship (e.g., *"I don't know why"*).

SUBTEST 5: DIGIT SPAN

Materials Test Form

Instructions Say, ***"I am going to say some numbers. Listen to the numbers, and when I finish, you say them back to me exactly the same way. Wait until I stop saying numbers before you begin."***

- Present numbers at the rate of 1 per second with even stress and prosody.
- Do not chunk numbers.
- No written responses are permitted on this subtest.

Discontinue Rule Discontinue if the child fails both sequences for any item and cross out scores for remaining items.

Repetition Not allowed

Scoring
- Cross out ability score for any incorrect item or for all items following discontinuation; circle ability score for each correct item.
- Add scores for correct items to compute total ability score.

Item	Stimuli/Responses	Ability Score	Item	Stimuli/Responses	Ability Score
1a	✓ ✓ *7 – 3*	(0.5)	1b	✓ ✓ *5 – 9*	(0.5)
2a	✓ ✓ ✓ *5 – 8 – 2*	(0.5)	2b	✓ ✓ ✓ *4 – 1 – 8*	(1.0)
3a	✓ ✓ ✓ ✓ *6 – 4 – 9 – 3*	(4.0)	3b	✓ ✓ ✓ ✓ *8 – 2 – 5 – 1*	(5.0)
4a	✓ ✓ ✓ ✓ ✓ *7 – 5 – 1 – 4 – 9*	(9.5)	4b	✓ ✓ ✓ ✓ ✓ *3 – 8 – 1 – 7 – 2*	(10.0)
5a	✓ ✓ ✓ ✓ ✓ ✓ *9 – 2 – 5 – 8 – 1 – 4*	(11.5)	5b	✓ ✓ ✓ ✓ ✓ ✓ *2 – 5 – 9 – 6 – 3 – 8*	(12.5)
6a	✓ ✓ ✓ ✓ ✓ ✓ *1 – 7 – 3 – 8 – 6 – ~~2~~ – 9*	~~13.5~~	6b	✓ ✓ ✓ ✓ ✓ ✓ ✓ *7 – 2 – 5 – 8 – 1 – 9 – 4*	(14.0)

Time to administer: 3 min. **Subtotal Score 1** 26.0 / 39.5

Subtotal Score 2 43.0 / 43.0
Subtotal Score 1 26.0 / 39.5
TOTAL DIGIT SPAN ABILITY SCORE 69.0 / 82.5

Behavioral observations: (Abbreviations may be used next to items where they apply.)

___ Repetition of instructions (Rep)	___ Perseveration (P)	___ No response (NR)
___ Attention reminder required (Attn)	___ Delayed response (5+ sec) (DR)	___ I don't know (IDK)
___ Prompt to reestablish set (Prompt)	___ Unintelligible response (UnR)	___ Self-correction (SC)

Additional qualitative/behavioral observations:

Immediate memory without processing demands remains a strength.

Notes for examiners on Digit Span: Digit Span is primarily a test of attention and immediate memory. In the early phase of recovery, Digit Span performance may be below normal range but then recover independently of tasks with higher level cognitive demands. You can examine qualitative patterns by writing the numbers as spoken by examinees. Look for patterns such as repeating correct numbers in the wrong order, remembering only first numbers (primacy) or last numbers (recency) in longer strings, substituting overlearned sequences (e.g., 3, 4, 5), and perseverating on numbers from earlier responses. Remember that this task requires verbal production of exact words and examinees are not allowed to write responses; therefore, it may not be a valid task for individuals who cannot speak.

NOTE: If you are administering this test in two sessions, end the first testing session here.

NOTE: *If you are administering this test in two sessions, start the second testing session here.*

SUBTEST 6: NAMING

Materials Test Form, Stimulus Book (page 11)

Instructions Open the Stimulus Book to page 11 and show the child the picture of the boy on his skateboard.
- Ask the child the question for each item in the table below while pointing to the precise location of the target item.
- If the child starts to elaborate, say, ***"Just give me one word."***

Record each response verbatim. If the child names an adjacent item, prompt, ***"No, this part."***
DO NOT tell the child to remember the picture for later

Discontinue Rule None

Repetition Repeat the question one time if the child does not respond within 10 seconds.

Scoring
- Cross out ability score for any incorrect item; circle ability score for each correct item.
- Add scores for correct items to compute total ability score.
- Do not penalize dysarthria or recognizable mispronunciations (e.g., *eblow*).

Item	Question	Target Item/Response	Ability Score
1	***What do you call these things?*** (If child names "trucks," [part of a skateboard], say, ***"No, this part,"*** and point again, specifically to wheels)	(Wheels)	(0.5)
2	***What do you call these things?*** (If child names "laces" [or other part], say, ***"No, the whole thing."***)	Boots / (Shoes)	(0.5)
3	***What do you call this thing?***	(Star)	(0.5)
4	***What do you call this thing?***	(Chain) / ID tags / Dog tags / Necklace	(1.5)
5	***What do you call this thing?***	(Band-Aid)	(2.0)
6	***What do you call this part of his body?***	(Chin)	(2.0)
7	***And this part of his body?***	(Elbow)	(2.5)
8	***And this part?*** (If child names "eye" [or other part], say, ***"No, this part."***)	(Eyebrow)	(3.0)

Time to administer: 2 min. **TOTAL NAMING ABILITY SCORE** 12.5 / 12.5

Behavioral observations: (Abbreviations may be used next to items where they apply.)

___ Repetition of instructions (Rep)	___ Perseveration (P)	___ No response (NR)
___ Attention reminder required (Attn)	___ Delayed response (5+ sec) (DR)	___ I don't know (IDK)
___ Prompt to reestablish set (Prompt)	___ Unintelligible response (UnR)	___ Self-correction (SC)

Additional qualitative/behavioral observations:

In contrast to Test 1, shows full recovery of ability to name these particular items.

Notes for examiners on Naming: Naming deficits are a key symptom of aphasia, and even delayed retrieval may be a sign of mild anomia. By recording an examinee's exact responses, you can identify error types such as semantic paraphasias (e.g., "ankle" for *elbow),* phonemic paraphasias (e.g., "eyetrow" for *eyebrow),* and circumlocutions (e.g., "put it around your neck" for *necklace/chain),* as well as perseverations. Look also for verbosity (elaboration rather than naming the item). In such cases, say, ***"Just give me one word."*** When misnaming occurs, try to identify the mechanism(s) for the error (e.g., language problem, visual acuity, visual perceptual deficits). In addition to testing naming ability, this subtest has a secondary purpose, which is to draw the examinee's attention to key elements of the picture for later recall (Subtest 9: Picture Recall). If the child comments on the danger of the skateboarder wearing a hat rather than a helmet, say, ***"You're absolutely right."***

SUBTEST 7: STORY RETELLING—IMMEDIATE

Materials Test Form, for children in: **Grades 1–3:** Read Story 1, "Bobby's Lucky Day."
Grades 4–7: Read Story 2, "Tommy the Trickster."
Grades 8–11: Read Story 3, "The Rock Concert."

Instructions Say, ***"I'm going to tell you a story. Listen carefully. I want you to repeat the whole story back to me exactly as I told it to you. I can only read it once. Are you ready?"*** Although "exactly" is in the instructions to the child, some semantically acceptable substitutions, as indicated, can receive credit.

"Okay, here is the story." Use natural inflection when reading the story.

After reading the story, say, ***"Now tell me the same story. Start now."***

Probe: If the child does not initiate the story, say, ***"What was the story about? What happened?"***

DO NOT tell the child to remember the story for later.

Discontinue Rule None

Repetition Repeat the directions one time if requested.
Prompt as indicated if the child does not begin retelling the story within 10 seconds.

Scoring

- Identify each correct story element recalled and circle corresponding ability score; cross out ability score for any omitted or incorrect item.
- Count acceptable semantic substitutions as correct.
- Do not count variations that change the meaning (e.g., "street" for *sidewalk*).
- Count pronouns as correct; but at first mention, the child must say characters' proper names (*Bobby, Tommy, Daryl, Rochelle).*
- Count elements told out of sequence as correct.
- Add scores for correct items to compute total ability score.

STORY 1 (GRADES 1–3)

Read the following story: "Bobby's Lucky Day"

"Bobby's grandmother gave him some money to buy candy. On his way to the store, the money fell out of a hole in his pocket. Bobby was really upset. But suddenly, he saw a dollar on the sidewalk in front of the store. It was Bobby's lucky day!"

Say, ***"Now tell me the same story. Start now."***

Probe: If the child does not initiate the story, say, ***"What was the story about? What happened?"***

Item	**Story Elements** (optional wording)	Ability Score	Item	**Story Elements** (optional wording)	Ability Score
1	Bobby's (must use proper name to count)	0.5	12	in his pocket	1.0
2	grandmother	2.0	13	Bobby (he)	3.0
3	gave him (Bobby)	1.5	14	(really) upset / mad	4.0
4	(some) money	1.0	15	but suddenly	5.5
5	to buy	3.0	16	he (Bobby) saw	1.5
6	candy	3.0	17	a dollar	1.0
7	on his way to	4.0	18	on the sidewalk	3.0
8	the store	3.0	19	in front of	3.0
9	(the) money	2.5	20	the store	2.5
10	fell out of	1.5	21	Bobby's (his)	1.5
11	a hole	2.0	22	lucky day	1.5

Time to administer: _____ **Subtotal Score 1** _____ / 24.0

Subtotal Score 2 _____ / 27.5

Subtotal Score 1 _____ / 24.0

TOTAL STORY RETELLING—IMMEDIATE ABILTY SCORE _____ / 51.5

STORY 3 (GRADES 8–11)

Read the following story: "The Rock Concert"

"Last spring, Daryl got two free tickets to an outdoor rock concert. So, he asked his friend Rochelle to go with him. Daryl said to his father, 'If you let me go to the concert with Rochelle and drive us there, I will take out the trash for three months.' Rochelle said to her mother, 'If you let me go to the concert with Daryl and pick us up afterwards, I promise to babysit my sister six times.' Both parents agreed. Ten minutes after the kids were dropped off, it began to pour. The concert was cancelled. The kids couldn't believe it. They would still have to keep their promises!"

Say, ***"Now tell me the same story. Start now."***

Probe: If the child does not initiate the story, say, ***"What was the story about? What happened?"***

Item	**Story Elements** (optional wording)	Ability Score	Item	**Story Elements** (optional wording)	Ability Score
1	Last spring *see below	~~4.5~~	23	months	~~2.5~~
2	Daryl got (must use proper name to count)	~~2.0~~	24	Rochelle (she) said	~~4.0~~
3	two	~~3.0~~	25	to her mother	~~4.0~~
4	free	~~4.0~~	26	if you let me go (allow me to go)	~~3.5~~
5	tickets to	~~1.5~~	27	and pick us up afterwards	~~1.0~~
6	outdoor	~~5.0~~	28	I promise	~~2.5~~
7	rock	~~2.5~~	29	to babysit	~~2.5~~
8	concert	~~0.5~~	30	my sister	~~5.0~~
9	so he asked	~~2.5~~	31	six times	~~5.0~~
10	his friend	~~3.0~~	32	both parents	~~5.0~~
11	Rochelle (must use proper name to count)	~~3.0~~	33	agreed	~~5.0~~
12	to go	~~3.5~~	34	ten	~~4.0~~
13	with him	~~4.0~~	35	minutes	~~3.5~~
14	Daryl (he) said	~~3.0~~	36	after the kids	~~1.0~~
15	to his father	~~2.0~~	37	were dropped off	~~2.5~~
16	if you let me go	~~3.0~~	38	it began to "pour" (rain)	~~2.0~~
17	to the concert	~~3.5~~	39	the concert	~~3.0~~
18	with Rochelle (her)	~~3.5~~	40	was cancelled	~~5.5~~
19	and drive us (there) (give us a ride)	~~4.0~~	41	the kids (they)	~~2.0~~
20	I will take out	~~2.0~~	42	couldn't believe it (**not**—they were mad)	~~5.5~~
21	the trash (garbage)	~~3.0~~	43	would still have to	~~2.0~~
22	three	~~2.5~~	44	keep their promises (do their jobs)	~~2.0~~

Time to administer: 6.5 min. **Subtotal Score 1** 0 / 65.5

Subtotal Score 2 0 / 73.0
Subtotal Score 1 0 / 65.5
TOTAL STORY RETELLING—IMMEDIATE ABILTY SCORE 0 / 138.5

* Said: "a little girl" "able to hold her"
"going" "country music"

Behavioral observations: (Abbreviations may be used next to items where they apply.)

___ Repetition of instructions (Rep)	___ Perseveration (P)	___ No response (NR)
___ Attention reminder required (Attn)	___ Delayed response (5+ sec) (DR)	___ I don't know (IDK)
___ Prompt to reestablish set (Prompt)	___ Unintelligible response (UnR)	___ Self-correction (SC)

Additional qualitative/behavioral observations:

Very poor performance on this test continues. Confabulatory story elements to fill memory gap. Weakest area at 5 months post. Need to address in therapy.

Note: Page 12 excluded because not relevant to this age range.

SUBTEST 8: YES/NO/MAYBE

Materials Test Form, Stimulus Book (pages 12–17)

Instructions Open the Stimulus Book to page 12 in front of the child.

Say, ***"Now we're going to read some very short stories together. I'll read and you follow along."*** (If the child can read aloud and wants to, let him or her do so. Do not require choral reading.)

Say, ***"Pay careful attention, because I'm going to ask you some questions after each story. Your answer can be 'yes' if you are certain the answer is 'yes,' or 'no' if you are certain the answer is 'no.' If the story doesn't clearly tell you the answer, you should say 'maybe.' Here is a practice item."***

- Do not remove the Stimulus Book; keep it in front of the child.
- Circle *Y* for "yes," *N* for "no," and *M* for "maybe" answers. Correct answers are in bold.

Note: If the child is unable to speak, write YES NO MAYBE in a vertical array on a piece of paper to allow a pointing response.

Discontinue Rule Discontinue testing if the child cannot get into set for the task after coaching on the practice story or if the child misses all items on two consecutive stories.

Repetition Only allowed during the practice story

Scoring
- Score self-corrections as correct only if immediate.
- Circle ability score for correct items; cross out ability score for incorrect items or items following discontinuation.
- Add subtotals for each short story.
- Compute total ability score by adding the story subscores.

Practice Story Say, ***"One morning, Susan missed the school bus. She thought she would be late for school, but her mother got her there on time."*** Say, ***"I can help you read it again if you want."***

Reread the story as often as requested, and then ask the following questions. Reinforce the correct answer for each practice question, and help the child to see the relationship if necessary.

a	***"Did Susan miss the bus?"***	(**Y**)	N	M
b	***"Was Susan late for school?"***	(Y)	**(N)**	M
c	***"Was it raining that morning?"***	Y	(N)	**(M)**
d	***"Did her father take her to school?"***	Y	(**N**)	M

Short Story 1 (Turn to page 13 in the Stimulus Book. *Note:* This story has only three questions.)

The kids ran after the blue ice cream truck. It turned the corner before they could catch it.

Item	Questions	Responses	Ability Score
a	***Did the kids chase the ice cream truck?***	(**Y**) N M	(0.5)
b	***Did the kids catch the truck before it turned the corner?***	Y (**N**) M	(0.5)
c	***Was the ice cream truck red?***	Y (**N**) M	(0.5)

Story 1 Ability Score 1.5 / 1.5

Short Story 2 (Turn to page 14 in the Stimulus Book.)

"What I did on my summer vacation" is the topic the teacher makes her class write about on the first day of school every year. When school started a month ago, the teacher gave her usual first writing assignment.

Item	Questions	Responses	Ability Score
a	***Did the teacher ask her class to write about their summer vacations?***	**(Y)** (N) M	~~0.5~~
b	***Was the Middle East the first writing topic of the year?***	Y (**N**) M	(3.5)
c	***Did school start last week?***	Y (**N**) M	(1.0)
d	***Did all of the students take a trip on their summer vacations?***	(Y) N **(M)**	~~2.0~~

Story 2 Ability Score 4.5 / 7.0
Story 1 Ability Score 1.5 / 1.5
Subtotal Score 6.0 / 8.5

Short Story 3 (Turn to page 15 in the Stimulus Book.)

Immanuel was the first one of a small group of boys in his class who could dunk a basketball.

Item	Questions	Responses	Ability Score
a	***Could Immanuel jump the highest in class?***	Y N **(M)** (circled)	1.0 (circled)
b	***Could some of the other boys dunk a basketball?***	**(Y)** (circled) N M	2.5 (circled)
c	***Could all of the boys in Immanuel's class dunk a basketball?***	Y **(N)** (circled) M	2.5 (circled)
d	***Was Immanuel the best basketball player in his class?***	Y N (circled) **(M)**	~~2.0~~

Story 3 Ability Score 6.0 / 8.0

Short Story 4 (Turn to page 16 in the Stimulus Book.)

Mary and Todd decided they would go to the beach on Saturday even if it was a cloudy day. When they woke up on Saturday, it was sunny.

Item	Questions	Responses	Ability Score
a	***Did Mary and Todd plan to go to the beach on Saturday if it was cloudy?***	**(Y)** N (circled) M	~~2.0~~
b	***Did it rain later on Saturday?***	Y N (circled) **(M)**	~~4.0~~
c	***Was it cloudy when Mary and Todd woke up on Saturday?***	Y **(N)** (circled) M	2.5 (circled)
d	***Was Mary the mother of Todd?***	Y N (circled) **(M)**	~~2.0~~

Story 4 Ability Score 2.5 / 10.5

Short Story 5 (Turn to page 17 in the Stimulus Book.)

The scientists observed the insects closely over a 24-hour period, hoping to study their swarming behavior. At that point, the scientists concluded that the insects had been prevented from swarming because of the unusual atmospheric conditions.

Item	Questions	Responses	Ability Score
a	***Did the insects swarm?***	Y (circled) **(N)** M	~~4.5~~
b	***Did the scientists watch the insects for a full day?***	**(Y)** (circled) N M	0.5 (circled)
c	***Can atmospheric conditions influence the swarming of insects?***	**(Y)** (circled) N M	2.5 (circled)
d	***Did the scientists accomplish their original goal?***	Y **(N)** (circled) M	4.5 (circled)

Time to administer: 6 min.

Story 5 Ability Score	7.5 / 12.0
Story 4 Ability Score	2.5 / 10.5
Story 3 Ability Score	6.0 / 8.0
Subtotal from page 14	6.0 / 8.5
TOTAL YES/NO/MAYBE ABILITY SCORE	22.0 / 39.0

Behavioral observations: (Abbreviations may be used next to items where they apply.)

___ Repetition of instructions (Rep)
___ Attention reminder required (Attn)
___ Prompt to reestablish set (Prompt)
✓ Perseveration (P)
___ Delayed response (5+ sec) (DR)
___ Unintelligible response (UnR)
___ No response (NR)
___ I don't know (IDK)
___ Self-correction (SC)

Additional qualitative/behavioral observations:
Unlike Test 1, now able to go through entire test. Perseverative responding greatly reduced. Notable improvement.

Notes for examiners on Yes/No/Maybe: The Yes/No/Maybe subtest was designed to test the ability to listen to/read short stories carefully enough to answer questions regarding both stated and inferred information. As such, this subtest requires several cognitive processes, including higher level language comprehension skills, attention, and mental tracking. In addition to computing the overall ability score, look for error patterns such as missing "maybe" responses or perseverating on one answer choice.

SUBTEST 9: PICTURE RECALL

Materials Test Form, Stimulus Book (page 11)

Instructions Say, ***"Remember the picture of the boy that I showed you a while ago?"*** If the child can't recall the picture, cue by saying, ***"The one where you named some parts of his body and other things."*** Then say, ***"Please draw that boy on this page."***

Use the last page of this Test Form.

Say, ***"Put in as many details as you can remember."***

Probe: If the child still can't remember the picture, say to the child, ***"Just draw a picture of any boy."***

When the child is finished or you see that he or she is not being productive, say, ***"Now we need your autograph. Please sign your first and last name on the bottom of your picture. Write it clearly so that anyone could read it."*** (Point to the bottom of the page.)

Probe: Okay to probe for last name if only first name is given.

Probe: If the picture is unclear or if the child is unable to draw, ask for a description, write down what the child says, and score recalled elements.

If the child cannot move to write his or her name, ask for a spelling. All letters in the name must be correct to receive credit.

Discontinue Rule If the child does not respond after 10 seconds following allowed prompting, discontinue.

Repetition If the child does not respond within 10 seconds, repeat the instructions and use the probe.

Scoring
- Circle ability score for any component recognizable in context.
- Cross out ability score for any missing component.
- All letters in name must be legible and correct for name to receive credit.
- Add subtotals for each column.
- Compute total ability score by adding the column subtotals.

Item	Picture Recall	Ability Score
1	Picture of a boy	(1.5)
2	Skateboard	~~3.0~~
3	Hat / Baseball cap	(5.5)
4	Boots / Shoes	(5.5)
5	Star	~~6.0~~
6	Chain / ID tags / Dog tags / Necklace	~~6.0~~
7	Band-Aid	~~7.0~~
8	Shorts	~~7.5~~

Picture Recall Subtotal 12.5 / 42.0

Item	Signature	Ability Score
1	First name	(0.5)
2	Last name	(3.0)

Signature Subtotal 3.5 / 3.5
Picture Recall Subtotal 12.5 /42.0
TOTAL PICTURE RECALL ABILITY SCORE 16.0 / 45.5

Time to administer: 6 min.

Hand used: ___ L ✓ R

Behavioral observations: (Abbreviations may be used next to items where they apply.)

___ Repetition of instructions (Rep)	___ Perseveration (P)	___ No response (NR)
___ Attention reminder required (Attn)	___ Delayed response (5+ sec) (DR)	___ I don't know (IDK)
___ Prompt to reestablish set (Prompt)	___ Unintelligible response (UnR)	___ Self-correction (SC)

Additional qualitative/behavioral observations:

Only slight improvement—recalls two details now. Again (see Story Retelling—Immediate) memory deficit is now most prominent problem.

Notes for examiners on Picture Recall: This subtest assesses incidental memory (i.e., without instruction to remember) for the picture presented in Subtest 6 and ability to depict recalled elements of that picture (through drawing, or speaking, in the case of individuals who are unable to hold a pen). The recalled components are scored, but it is important that you study the picture carefully and look for such features as micrographia (tiny drawing), proportionality, perseverative elements, unilateral neglect (drawing only half the picture), and fragmentation (refer to the *PTBI Examiner's Manual* for examples). Signatures as well as spelling can be analyzed for some of these same features.

SUBTEST 10: STORY RETELLING—DELAYED

Materials Test Form, for children in:
Grades 1–3: Score Story 1, "Bobby's Lucky Day."
Grades 4–7: Score Story 2, "Tommy the Trickster."
Grades 8–11: Score Story 3, "The Rock Concert."

Instructions Do not reread the story. The child must recall the story from the prior experience.

Say, ***"Remember the story [title of story child heard]? Tell me the story again. Try to remember as much as you can."***

As the child retells the story, check story elements recalled correctly or record verbatim any content variations in the story produced.

Discontinue Rule None

Repetition Repeat the directions one time if requested.

Scoring

- Identify each correct story element recalled and circle corresponding ability score; cross out ability score for any omitted or incorrect item.
- Count acceptable semantic substitutions as correct.
- Do not count variations that change the meaning (e.g., "street" for *sidewalk*).
- Count pronouns as correct; but at first mention, the child must say characters' proper names (*Bobby, Tommy, Daryl, Rochelle*).
- Count elements told out of sequence as correct.
- Add scores for correct items to compute total ability score.

STORY 1 (GRADES 1–3)

Say, ***"Remember the story 'Bobby's Lucky Day'? Tell me the story again. Try to remember as much as you can"***

Item	**Story Elements** (optional wording)	Ability Score
1	Bobby's (must use proper name to count)	1.5
2	grandmother	1.5
3	gave him (Bobby)	1.5
4	(some) money	1.5
5	to buy	3.5
6	candy	3.5
7	on his way to	4.0
8	the store	3.0
9	(the) money	2.0
10	fell out of	1.5
11	a hole	2.0

Time to administer: _____ **Subtotal Score 1** _____ / 25.5

Item	**Story Elements** (optional wording)	Ability Score
12	in his pocket	1.0
13	Bobby (he)	3.5
14	(really) upset / mad	4.5
15	but suddenly	5.5
16	he (Bobby) saw	0.5
17	a dollar	0.5
18	on the sidewalk	3.0
19	in front of	3.5
20	the store	2.5
21	Bobby's (his)	2.0
22	lucky day	2.0

Subtotal Score 2 _____ / 28.5

Subtotal Score 1 _____ / 25.5

TOTAL STORY RETELLING—DELAYED ABILTY SCORE _____ / 51.5

STORY 3 (GRADES 8–11)

Say. ***Remember the story 'The Rock Concert'? Tell me the story again. Try to remember as much as you can."***

Item	**Story Elements** (optional wording)	Ability Score	Item	**Story Elements** (optional wording)	Ability Score
1	Last spring **see below*	~~4.0~~	23	months	~~2.5~~
2	Daryl got (must use proper name to count)	~~2.0~~	24	Rochelle (she) said	~~2.5~~
3	two	~~2.5~~	25	to her mother	~~1.5~~
4	free	~~4.0~~	26	if you let me go (allow me to go)	~~3.0~~
5	tickets to	~~1.0~~	27	and pick us up afterwards	~~3.0~~
6	outdoor	~~4.5~~	28	I promise	~~2.5~~
7	rock	~~1.5~~	29	to babysit	~~1.0~~
8	concert	~~0.5~~	30	my sister	~~2.5~~
9	so he asked	~~2.0~~	31	six times	~~2.5~~
10	his friend	~~2.5~~	32	both parents	~~4.0~~
11	Rochelle (must use proper name to count)	~~2.5~~	33	agreed	~~3.5~~
12	to go	~~2.5~~	34	ten	~~3.5~~
13	with him	~~3.5~~	35	minutes	~~3.5~~
14	Daryl (he) said	~~2.5~~	36	after the kids	~~3.0~~
15	to his father	~~1.5~~	37	were dropped off	~~3.0~~
16	if you let me go	~~3.0~~	38	it began to "pour" (rain)	~~1.0~~
17	to the concert	~~4.0~~	39	the concert	~~1.0~~
18	with Rochelle (her)	~~4.5~~	40	was cancelled	~~1.5~~
19	and drive us (there) (give us a ride)	~~3.0~~	41	the kids (they)	~~3.0~~
20	I will take out	~~1.5~~	42	couldn't believe it [**not**—they were mad]	~~3.5~~
21	the trash (garbage)	~~1.0~~	43	would still have to	~~1.5~~
22	three	~~2.5~~	44	keep their promises (do their jobs)	~~1.5~~

Time to administer: *3 min.* **Subtotal Score 1** *0* / 56.5

**Said, "They had a brother and sister and needed everyone to keep on him."*

Subtotal Score 2 *0* / 54.5
Subtotal Score 1 *0* / 56.5
TOTAL STORY RETELLING—DELAYED ABILTY SCORE *0* / 111.0

Behavioral observations: (Abbreviations may be used next to items where they apply.)

___ Repetition of instructions (Rep)	✓ Perseveration (P)	___ No response (NR)
___ Attention reminder required (Attn)	___ Delayed response (5+ sec) (DR)	___ I don't know (IDK)
___ Prompt to reestablish set (Prompt)	___ Unintelligible response (UnR)	___ Self-correction (SC)

Additional qualitative/behavioral observations:

Different confabulated info compared with that of immediate recall condition. Not encoding information in immediate condition for recall in delayed condition.

Note: Page 18 excluded because not relevant to this age range.

SUBTEST 9: PICTURE RECALL

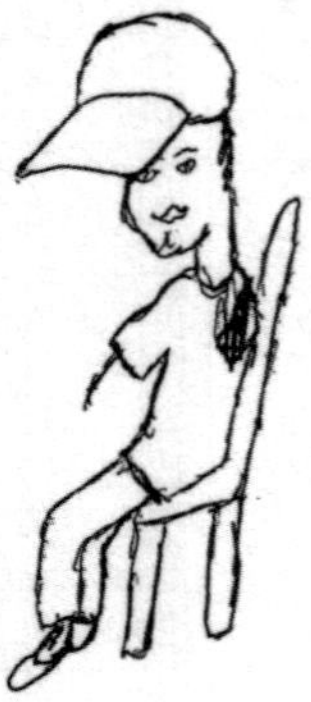

References

Adelson, P.D., Bratton, S.I., Carney, N.A., Chestnut, R.M., du Coudray, E.M., Goldstein, B., et al. (2003). Guidelines for the acute medical management of severe traumatic brain injury in infants, children and adolescents. *Pediatric Critical Care Medicine, 4*(Suppl. 3), S2–S35.

American Educational Research Association/American Psychological Association/National Council on Measurement in Education. (1999). *Standards for educational and psychological testing.* Washington, DC: American Psychological Association.

American Speech-Language-Hearing Association. (2003). *Rehabilitation of children and adults with cognitive-communication disorders after brain injury.* [Technical Report]. Available at http://www.asha.org/policy

Anastasi, A., & Urbina, S. (1997). *Psychological testing* (7th ed.). New York: Macmillan.

Angoff, W.H., & Ford, S.F. (1973). Item-race interactions on a test of scholastic ability. *Journal of Educational Measurement, 10,* 95–106.

Babikian, T., & Asarnow, R. (2009). Neurocognitive outcomes and recovery after pediatric TBI: Meta-analytical review of the literature. *Neuropsychology, 3*(3), 283–296.

Bedore, L.M., Peña, E.D., García, M., & Cortez, C. (2005). Conceptual versus monolingual scoring: When does it make a difference? *Language, Speech, & Hearing Services in Schools, 36,* 188–200.

Chapman, S.B., Levin, H.S., Wanek A., Weyrach, J., & Kufera, J.A. (1998). Discourse after closed head injury in children. *Brain & Language, 61*(3), 420–449.

Cicerone, K.D. (1996). Attention deficits and dual task demands after mild traumatic brain injury. *Brain Injury, 10,* 79–89.

Crosson, B., Novack, T., Trenerry, M.S., & Cragi, L.P. (1988). California Verbal Learning Test (CVLT) performance in severely head injured and neurologically normal adult males. *Journal of Clinical and Experimental Neuropsychology, 10,* 754–768.

Ewing-Cobbs, L., Levin, H.S., Eisenberg, H.M., & Fletcher, J.M. (1987). Language functions following closed head injury in children and adolescents. *Journal of Clinical and Experimental Neuropsychology, 9,* 575–592.

Ewing-Cobbs, L., Miner, M.E., Fletcher, J.M., & Levin, H.S. (1989). Intellectual motor and language sequelae following closed head injury in infants and preschoolers. *Journal of Pediatric Psychology, 14,* 531–547.

Fay, T.B., Yeates, K.O., Wade, S.L., Drotar, D., Stancin, T., & Taylor, G.H. (2009). Predicting longitudinal patterns of functional deficits in children with traumatic brain injury. *Neuropsychology, 23*(3), 271–182.

Goldstein, F.C., Len, H.S., & Boake, C. (1989). Conceptual encoding following severe closed head injury. *Cortex, 25,* 541–554.

Gollan, T.H., & Kroll, J.F. (2001). Bilingual lexical access. In B. Rapp (Ed.), *The handbook of cognitive neuropsychology: What deficits reveal about the human mind* (pp. 321–345). Philadelphia: Psychology Press.

Gulliksen, H. (1950). *Theory of mental tests.* New York: John Wiley & Sons.

Hagen, C., Malkmus, D., & Durham, P. (1979). *Levels of cognitive functioning: Rehabilitation of the head injured adult. Comprehensive, physical management.* Downey, CA: Professional Staff Association, Rancho Los Amigos Hospital.

Hartley, L., (1995). *Cognitive communicative abilities following brain injury: A functional approach.* San Diego: Singular.

Hotz, G., Helm-Estabrooks, N., & Nelson, N.W. (2001). Development of the Pediatric Test of Brain Injury. *Journal of Head Trauma Rehabilitation, 16*(5), 426–440.

Hotz, G., Helm-Estabrooks, N., Nelson, N.W., & Plante, E. (2009). The Pediatric Test of Brain Injury: Development and interpretation. *Topics in Language Disorders, 29*(3), 207–223.

Jantz, P.B., & Coulter, G.A. (2007). Traumatic brain injury. Child and adolescent traumatic brain injury: Academic, behavioural, and social consequences in the classroom. *Support for Learning, 22*(2), 84–89.

Krichevsky, M., Chang, J., & Squire, L.R. (2004). Functional amnesia: Clinical description and neuropsychological profile of 10 cases. *Learning and Memory, 11*, 213–226.

Levin, H.S., Culhane, K.A., Mendelsohn, D., Lilly, M.A., Bruce, D., Fletcher, J.M., et al. (1993). Cognition in relation to magnetic resonance imaging in head injured children and adolescents. *Archives of Neurology, 50*, 897–905.

Levin, H.S., Fletcher, J.M., Kusnerick, L., Kufera J.A., Lilly, M.A., Duffy, F., et al. (1996). Semantic memory following pediatric head injury: Relationship to age, severity of injury and MRI. *Cortex, 32*(3), 461–478.

Levin, H.S., Hanten, G., Zhang, L., Swank, P.R., Ewing-Cobbs, L., Dennis, M., et al. (2004). Changes in working memory after traumatic brain injury in children. *Neuropsychology, 18*(2), 240–247.

Levin, H.S., Song, J., Scheibel, R.S., Fletcher, J.M., Harward, H., Lilly, M., et al. (1997). Concept formation and problem-solving following closed head injury in children. *Journal of the International Neuropsychological Society, 3*, 598–607.

Lezak, M.D., Howieson, D.B., Loring, D.W., Hannay, H.J., & Fisher, J.S. (2004). *Neuropsychological assessment* (4th ed.). New York: Oxford University Press.

McDowell, S., Whyte, J., & D'Esposito, M. (1997). Working memory impairments in traumatic brain injury: Evidence from a dual-task paradigm. *Neuropsychologia, 35*(10), 134–153.

McKay, K.E., Halperin, J.M., Schwartz, S.T., & Sharma, V. (1994). Developmental analysis of three aspects of information processing: Sustained attention, selective attention, and response organization. *Developmental Neuropsychology, 10*, 121–132.

Michael, E.B., & Gollan, T.H. (2005). Being and becoming bilingual: Individual differences and consequences for language production. In J.F. Kroll & A.M.B. de Groot (Eds.), *Handbook of bilingualism: Psycholinguistic approaches* (pp. 389–407). New York: Oxford University Press.

Milton, S.B., Scaglione, C., Flanagan, T., Cox, J.L., & Rudnick, D.F. (1991). Functional evaluation of adolescent student with traumatic brain injury. *Journal of Head Trauma Rehabilitation*, 6, 35–46.

Paris, S.G. (2005). Reinterpreting the development of reading skills. *Reading Research Quarterly, 40*, 184–202.

Portocarrero, J.S., Burright, R.G., & Donovick, P.J. (2007). Vocabulary and verbal fluency of bilingual and monolingual college students. *Archives of Clinical Neuropsychology, 22*, 415–422.

Rao, V., & Lyketsos, C. (2000). Neuropsychiatric sequelae of traumatic brain injury. *Psychosomatics, 41*(2), 95–103.

Raskin, S.A., Mateer, C.A., & Tweeten, R. (1998). Neuropsychological assessment of individuals with mild traumatic brain injury. *The Clinical Neuropsychologist, 12*, 21–30.

Slomine, B.S., Gering, J.P., Grados, M.A., Vasa, R., Brady, K.D., Christensen, J.R., et al. (2002). Performance on measures of "executive function" following pediatric traumatic brain injury. *Brain Injury, 16*(9), 759–772.

Stein, N., & Glenn, C.G. (1982). Children's concept of time: The development of a story schema. In W. Freeman (Ed.), *The developmental psychology of time* (pp. 255–282). Norwood, NJ: Ablex.

Stuss, D.S., (1991). Self-awareness and the frontal lobes: A neuropsychological prospective. In G.R. Goethals and J. Strauss (Eds.), *The self: An interdisciplinary approach* (pp. 255–278). New York: Springer-Verlag.

Teasdale, G., & Jennett, B. (1974). Assessment of Coma and Impaired Consciousness: A practical scale. *Lancet, 2*, 81–84.

Vital, M. (2002).*Traumatic brain injury: Hope through research* (NIH Pub. No. 02-158). Bethesda, MD: National Institute of Neurological Disorders and Stroke.

Westby, C.E. (1994). The effects of culture on genre, structure, and style of oral and written texts. In G.P. Wallach & K.G. Butler (Eds.), *Language-learning disabilities in school-age children and adolescents* (pp. 180–218). Boston: Allyn & Bacon.

Wilde, M.C., Boake, C., & Sherer, M. (1995). Do recognition free recall discrepancies detect retrieval deficits in closed head injury? An exploratory analysis with California Verbal Learning Test. *Journal of Clinical and Experimental Neuropsychology, 17*, 849–855.

Ylvisaker, M. (Ed.). (1998). *Traumatic brain injury rehabilitation: Children and adolescents.* Boston: Butterworth-Heinemann.

Ylvisaker, M., Adelson, P.D., Braga, L.W., Burnett, S.M., Glang, A., & Feeney, T. (2005). Rehabilitation and ongoing support after pediatric TBI: Twenty years of progress. *Journal of Head Trauma Rehabilitation, 20*(1), 95–109.

A

Appendix

Performance Categories Based on Age

PERFORMANCE CATEGORIES: AGE 6

	Very low performance	Low performance	Moderate performance	High performance
1. Orientation	0–9	9.5–18	18.5–25.5	26–38
2. Following Commands	0–11	11.5–12.5	13–14.5	15
3. Word Fluency	0–3	4–6	7–15	16 or more
4. What Goes Together	0–15.5	16–24.5	25–41.5	42–100.5
5. Digit Span	0	0.5–7.5	8–20.5	21–82.5
6. Naming	0–9.5	10–11.5	12	12.5
7. Story Retelling—Immediate				
Story 1	0–5	5.5–11.5	12–22.5	23–51.5
8. Yes/No/Maybe	0–4	4.5–9.5	10–14	14.5–39
9. Picture Recall	0–2	2.5–14.5	15–24.5	25–45.5
10. Story Retelling—Delayed				
Story 1	0–2.5	3–10.5	11–21.5	22–54

PERFORMANCE CATEGORIES: AGE 7

	Very low performance	Low performance	Moderate performance	High performance
1. Orientation	0–14	14.5–31	31.5–37.5	38
2. Following Commands	0–11	11.5–12.5	13–14.5	15
3. Word Fluency	0–5	6–11	12–19	20 or more
4. What Goes Together	0–12.5	13–24.5	25–41.5	42–100.5
5. Digit Span	0	0.5–7.5	8–20	21–82.5
6. Naming	0–10.5	11–11.5	12	12.5
7. Story Retelling—Immediate				
Story 1	0–4.5	5–11.5	12–22.5	23–51.5
8. Yes/No/Maybe	0–5	5.5–10	10.5–16.5	17–39
9. Picture Recall	0–5	5.5–17.5	18–27	27.5–45.5
10. Story Retelling—Delayed				
Story 1	0–2.5	3–10.5	11–21.5	22–54

PERFORMANCE CATEGORIES: AGE 8

	Very low performance	Low performance	Moderate performance	High performance
1. Orientation	0–17	17.5–32.5	33–37.5	38
2. Following Commands	0–10.5	11–14.5	—	15
3. Word Fluency	0–9	10–20	21–25	26 or more
4. What Goes Together	0–17.5	18–29.5	30–51.5	52–100.5
5. Digit Span	0	0.5–7.5	8–24	24.5–82.5
6. Naming	0–10.5	11–11.5	12	12.5
7. Story Retelling—Immediate[a]				
Story 1	0–4	4.5–11.5	12–22.5	23–51.5
Story 2	0–33	33.5–66	66.5–80.5	81–142.5
8. Yes/No/Maybe	0–4.5	5–10.5	11–17.5	18–39
9. Picture Recall	0–10	10.5–19	19.5–30.5	31–45.5
10. Story Retelling—Delayed[a]				
Story 1	0–3.5	4–10.5	11–21.5	22–54
Story 2	0–19.5	20–32.5	33–40	40.5–83

[a]Only one story is administered per child. Stories are assigned by grade level.

PERFORMANCE CATEGORIES: AGE 9

	Very low performance	Low performance	Moderate performance	High performance
1. Orientation	0–29.5	30–37.5	–	38
2. Following Commands	0–10.5	11–14.5	–	15
3. Word Fluency	0–9	10–20	21–25	26 or more
4. What Goes Together	0–19.5	20–39.5	40–59.5	60–100.5
5. Digit Span	0–6	6.5–18	18.5–25.5	26–82.5
6. Naming	0–10	10.5–11.5	12	12.5
7. Story Retelling—Immediate[a]				
Story 1	0–4	4.5–11.5	12–22.5	23–51.5
Story 2	0–33	33.5–66	66.5–80.5	81–142.5
8. Yes/No/Maybe	0–6.5	7–12	12.5–17.5	18–39
9. Picture Recall	0–10	10.5–21.5	22–30.5	31–45.5
10. Story Retelling—Delayed[a]				
Story 1	0–3.5	4–10.5	11–21.5	22–54
Story 2	0–19.5	20–32.5	33–40	40.5–83

[a]Only one story is administered per child. Stories are assigned by grade level.

PERFORMANCE CATEGORIES: AGE 10

	Very low performance	Low performance	Moderate performance	High performance
1. Orientation	0–29.5	30–37.5	–	38
2. Following Commands	0–10.5	11–14.5	–	15
3. Word Fluency	0–10	11–22	23–29	30 or more
4. What Goes Together	0–24.5	25–49.5	50–73.5	74–100.5
5. Digit Span	0–6	6.5–17.5	18–28	28.5–82.5
6. Naming	0–10	10.5–12	–	12.5
7. Story Retelling—Immediate[a]				
Story 1	0–4	4.5–11.5	12–22.5	23–51.5
Story 2	0–33	33.5–66	66.5–80.5	81–142.5
8. Yes/No/Maybe	0–8.5	9–14	14.5–19.5	20–39
9. Picture Recall	0–15.5	16–25.5	26–31.5	32–45.5
10. Story Retelling—Delayed[a]				
Story 1	0–7.5	8–10.5	11–21.5	22–54
Story 2	0–15.5	16–23.5	24–43	43.5–83

[a]Only one story is administered per child. Stories are assigned by grade level.

PERFORMANCE CATEGORIES: AGE 11

	Very low performance	Low performance	Moderate performance	High performance
1. Orientation	0–29.5	30–37.5	–	38
2. Following Commands	0–10.5	11–14.5	–	15
3. Word Fluency	0–12	13–23	24–30	31 or more
4. What Goes Together	0–24.5	25–49.5	50–74.5	75–100.5
5. Digit Span	0–9.5	10–19.5	20–30.5	31–82.5
6. Naming	0–10	10.5–12	–	12.5
7. Story Retelling—Immediate Story 2	0–33	33.5–66	66.5–80.5	81–142.5
8. Yes/No/Maybe	0–10.5	11–16	16.5–21.5	22–39
9. Picture Recall	0–15.5	16–27.5	28–33.5	34–45.5
10. Story Retelling—Delayed Story 2	0–15.5	16–23.5	24–43	43.5–83

PERFORMANCE CATEGORIES: AGE 12

	Very low performance	Low performance	Moderate performance	High performance
1. Orientation	0–29.5	30–37.5	–	38
2. Following Commands	0–10.5	11–14.5	–	15
3. Word Fluency	0–10	11–23	24–31	32 or more
4. What Goes Together	0–24.5	25–49.5	50–75.5	76–100.5
5. Digit Span	0–11.5	12–23.5	24–34.5	35–82.5
6. Naming	0–10	10.5–12	–	12.5
7. Story Retelling—Immediate[a]				
Story 2	0–33	33.5–66	66.5–80.5	81–142.5
Story 3	0–29.5	30–62	62.5–81.5	82–138.5
8. Yes/No/Maybe	0–11.5	12–18.5	19–23	23.5–39
9. Picture Recall	0–19	19.5–29.5	30–36	36.5–45.5
10. Story Retelling—Delayed[a]				
Story 2	0–15.5	16–23.5	24–43	43.5–83
Story 3	0–25.5	26–56.5	57–81	81.5–111

[a]Only one story is administered per child. Stories are assigned by grade level.

PERFORMANCE CATEGORIES: AGE 13

	Very low performance	Low performance	Moderate performance	High performance
1. Orientation	0–29.5	30–37.5	–	38
2. Following Commands	0–10.5	11–14.5	–	15
3. Word Fluency	0–11	12–25	26–31	32 or more
4. What Goes Together	0–24.5	25–49.5	50–76.5	77–100.5
5. Digit Span	0–11.5	12–23.5	24–34.5	35–82.5
6. Naming	0–10	10.5–12	–	12.5
7. Story Retelling—Immediate[a]				
Story 2	0–33	33.5–66	66.5–80.5	81–142.5
Story 3	0–29.5	30–49.5	50–70.5	71–138.5
8. Yes/No/Maybe	0–15.5	16–20.5	21–25	25.5–39
9. Picture Recall	0–24	24.5–32.5	33–37.5	38–45.5
10. Story Retelling—Delayed[a]				
Story 2	0–15.5	16–23.5	24–43	43.5–83
Story 3	0–21.5	22–35	35.5–45	45.5–111

[a]Only one story is administered per child. Stories are assigned by grade level.

PERFORMANCE CATEGORIES: AGE 14

	Very low performance	Low performance	Moderate performance	High performance
1. Orientation	0–29.5	30–37.5	–	38
2. Following Commands	0–10.5	11–14.5	–	15
3. Word Fluency	0–11	12–25	26–31	32 or more
4. What Goes Together	0–24.5	25–49.5	50–79.5	80–100.5
5. Digit Span	0–13.5	14–24.5	25–37.5	38–82.5
6. Naming	0–10	10.5–12	–	12.5
7. Story Retelling—Immediate[a]				
Story 2	0–33	33.5–66	66.5–80.5	81–142.5
Story 3	0–29.5	30–49.5	50–70.5	71–138.5
8. Yes/No/Maybe	0–14.5	15–20	20.5–25.5	26–39
9. Picture Recall	0–25	25.5–33.5	34–38.5	39–45.5
10. Story Retelling—Delayed[a]				
Story 2	0–15.5	16–23.5	24–43	43.5–83
Story 3	0–21.5	22–35	35.5–45	45.5–111

[a]Only one story is administered per child. Stories are assigned by grade level.

PERFORMANCE CATEGORIES: AGE 15

	Very low performance	Low performance	Moderate performance	High performance
1. Orientation	0–29.5	30–37.5	—	38
2. Following Commands	0–10.5	11–14.5	—	15
3. Word Fluency	0–11	12–25	26–31	32 or more
4. What Goes Together	0–37.5	38–69.5	70–81.5	82–100.5
5. Digit Span	0–18.5	19–29.5	30–41.5	42–82.5
6. Naming	0–10	10.5–12	—	12.5
7. Story Retelling—Immediate				
Story 3	0–29.5	30–49.5	50–70.5	71–138.5
8. Yes/No/Maybe	0–14.5	15–20.5	21–25.5	26–39
9. Picture Recall	0–25	25.5–33.5	34–38.5	39–45.5
10. Story Retelling—Delayed				
Story 3	0–31.5	32–45	45.5–55	55.5–111

PERFORMANCE CATEGORIES: AGE 16

	Very low performance	Low performance	Moderate performance	High performance
1. Orientation	0–29.5	30–37.5	–	38
2. Following Commands	0–10.5	11–14.5	–	15
3. Word Fluency	0–11	12–26	27–32	33 or more
4. What Goes Together	0–37.5	38–75.5	76–81.5	82–100.5
5. Digit Span	0–23.5	24–37.5	38–49.5	50–82.5
6. Naming	0–10	10.5–12	–	12.5
7. Story Retelling—Immediate				
Story 3	0–29.5	30–62	62.5–81.5	82–138.5
8. Yes/No/Maybe	0–14.5	15–20.5	21–25.5	26–39
9. Picture Recall	0–25	25.5–33.5	34–38.5	39–45.5
10. Story Retelling—Delayed				
Story 3	0–29.5	30–45	45.5–59.5	60–111

B

Appendix

Standard Error of Measurement by Subtest and Age

Subtest	Age (years)										
	6	7	8	9	10	11	12	13	14	15	16
1. Orientation	3	2	2	1	1	0	0	0	0	0	0
2. Following Commands	0	0	0	0	0	0	0	0	0	0	0
3. Word Fluency	2	3	4	4	3	3	4	4	6	4	2
4. What Goes Together	4	10	11	11	10	8	8	8	13	10	6
5. Digit Span	9	8	7	4	9	8	5	5	10	3	4
6. Naming	0	0	0	0	0	0	0	0	0	0	0
7. Story Retelling—Immediate											

Story 1	6	6	6	6	6	6	—	—	—	—	—
Story 2	—	—	14	14	14	14	14	14	14	—	—
Story 3	—	—	—	—	—	—	13	13	13	13	13
8. Yes/No/Maybe	3	2	2	2	3	3	2	3	3	2	2
9. Picture Recall	5	5	4	5	2	3	3	3	2	3	2
10. Story Retelling—Delayed											
Story 1	6	6	6	6	6	6	—	—	—	—	—
Story 2	—	—	7	7	7	7	7	7	7	—	—
Story 3	—	—	—	—	—	—	7	7	7	7	7

These values were based on test–retest reliability data obtained with children without brain injuries (see Table 6.8). Therefore, the values reflect the amount of score variability likely to occur from one test session to another in children whose neurological status is assumed to be stable.

Index

Tables and figures are indicated by *t* and *f*, respectively.